DALE PINNOCK The MEDICINAL CHEF

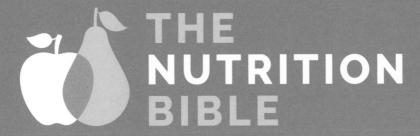

THE NUTRITION BIBLE

An A–Z of ailments and medicinal foods

Hardie Grant

QUADRILLE

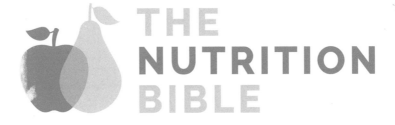

THE
NUTRITION
BIBLE

Publishing Director: Sarah Lavelle
Senior Commissioning Editor: Céline Hughes
Head of Design: Claire Rochford
Design: Jim Smith
Head of Production: Stephen Lang
Production Controller: Katie Jarvis

First published in 2020 by Quadrille Publishing,
an imprint of Hardie Grant Publishing

Quadrille
52–54 Southwark Street
London SE1 1UN
quadrille.com

Text © Dale Pinnock 2020
Design and layout © Quadrille Publishing 2020

ISBN: 978 1 78713 251 1

Printed in China

Contents

Introduction

There is no escaping the fact that nutrition has become big business – huge, in fact. Wherever we are, we seem to be exposed to swathes of information about diet and lifestyle. From aspirational images of avocado toast and green drinks on social media, through to scare stories about the dangers of every conceivable food in our newspapers, we are bombarded. We see hosts of young 'gurus' telling us the way we should eat and seeking to inspire us; and some of them barely seem to be older than teenagers! We are lost in a sea of opinion from a multitude of people many of whom do not have the qualifications to give advice in this complex and often contradictory and divisive subject. We are utterly bombarded and this has brought with it confusion and, in some cases, overt scepticism – all of which is understandable.

However, I firmly believe that it is vital that we get to grips with the fundamentals of nutrition. It is the cornerstone of our health. I personally feel that nutrition and lifestyle represent one aspect of our health care that we can actively engage in. We can take conscious, determined steps to safeguard our health in both the short term and the long term.

The truth is that the nutrients in the food that we eat directly influence the internal biochemical terrain of our bodies. From energy and repair, through to the most intricate of intra- and extracellular reactions and responses, elements of our diet are involved. Carbohydrates and fats give us energy. Fats help to build cells and hormones. Protein helps the body to repair damaged or stressed tissues and provides the building blocks for our own proteins, which play thousands of different roles in the body. Vitamins and minerals work as chemical cofactors that make reactions happen. Some minerals help cells to communicate. You get the idea.

Our diet is so fundamentally vital to our health that it simply cannot be ignored.

With almost 26 years in the industry, I have made it my mission to provide clarity and understanding in this realm. If you can get to grips with the basics – the need-to-knows and key fundamentals – then you can take steps, every day, to protect your health.

On top of these fundamentals, having reliable resources on hand to access key pieces of information when you need them gives you valuable tools for a healthy future. That's what this book is here to do.

Many of you will know me for creating books that break down the science around delicious, nutritious recipes. This is my first ever deviation from that format because for a long time I have felt that there needs to be a clear and straightforward reference book on all things nutrition. The problem with trawling through the internet for answers is that you are in essence trawling through endless unfiltered, unsupported opinions. I'm here to provide a very simple evidence-based reference for you in a user-friendly package.

In this book, you will find sections on the key nutritional needs and focus points for different life stages. You will find information on what ailments can be positively impacted by nutritional intervention, and what different everyday foods and ingredients do and how. There is also a section on one of the most hotly debated and researched areas of nutrition – supplementation.

I hope this becomes a go-to resource for you and your family when you want to separate the facts from fiction.

Nutrition Through the Life Stages

Nutrition is one of the most important subjects that you can familiarize yourself with. It is the foundation of good health from the moment you are a growing foetus. Most people see food as simply fuel, which partially it is, but food – and by extension nutrition – is way more than that. Indeed, it can completely influence our bodies' processes. It affects thousands of chemical reactions within our cells, including how tissues and structures grow and develop, how resilient these become to damage, whether systems thrive or become diseased and more. Good nutrition can have the power to keep you going to a ripe old age; bad nutrition to take you in your prime. Our diet is important: make no mistake about that. Taking time to learn about this vital subject could actually save the lives of you and your family and keep you all in good health for generations.

While some of the rules of the game stay the same for a lifetime, there are variations in nutritional needs at different stages of our lives. For example, the requirements of a teenager versus those of the elderly can vary greatly. So, with that in mind, one of the best places to start is to learn about the changing nutritional needs that we have as we progress through life.

Nutrition during infancy and weaning

Human beings grow faster in the first year of life than at any other time. A baby's growth is especially related to nutritional status. The baby's birthweight doubles at around four months and triples by the time they reach one year. During this rapid growth stage, breast milk and formula are the order of the day to supply the high concentrations of the growth nutrients babies need, such as proteins and fats and key minerals like iron and calcium. Once the infant begins to move towards solid foods, it is essential to try to get key vitamins and minerals into their diet.

Iron

Iron is an important nutrient at any age, and a mineral that can commonly be deficient in infants. It plays a vital role in haematopoiesis – the manufacture of blood cells. It is also a key part in haemoglobin. This is a protein complex found on each red blood cell that binds oxygen to it to take it around the body to our cells and tissues. It is a structure of four unique proteins bound together, at the centre of which sits iron. Oxygen binds to this iron and piggybacks on to it to be taken around the body to the cells and tissues that demand it. This is why low iron levels cause low energy – less oxygen is delivered around the body for all of its vital functions to be performed, for muscles to do their job, etc. Iron is also important for the production of enzymes, the manufacture of new cells and production of important substances such as amino acids and hormones.

You can see why iron is important for all of us, but in a tiny body that is growing at a rate of knots, many of these functions are heightened. Lower-than-adequate levels of iron in babies can cause deficits and slowing of cognitive and behavioural development, so iron should be a high priority during weaning.

BEST SOURCES OF IRON-RICH FOODS
- Red meats such as beef, pork, lamb, etc.
- Poultry
- Eggs
- Beans and pulses (legumes)
- Dark green, leafy vegetables

TIP: Add vitamin C-rich foods alongside iron-rich foods, as vitamin C increases iron absorption.

Omega-3 fatty acids

Fatty acids are fat-derived compounds that have a vitamin-like nature in that they are essential for regulating biochemical activities in the body, and they also have a structural role to play. Essential fatty acids are 'essential' because the body cannot manufacture them itself, so we need to get them from our diet.

There are several families of omega fatty acids: omega-3, omega-6, omega-7 and omega-9. Of all these, the omega-3 are the most important during infant and child development and, in my opinion, throughout the entire lifespan.

In the developing infant, omega-3 fatty acids play a *vital* role in the development of brain and nervous tissues. Our brain is made up of at least 60% fat, with up to 30% of this being omega-3 fatty acids. These fats make up the outer casing of nerve cells that are essential for rapidly and effectively conveying signals throughout the brain and nervous system. Our nerve cells are very long cells that can sometimes run as far as the distance of half the body. This system carries information in the form of electrical impulses. If these impulses were to travel along the nerve cell at a regular pace, the signals would take a long time (fractions of a second, but a long time in nervous conduction terms) to get where they are going and deliver the intended response. Because of this, nerve cells need a special way to send these messages faster than the speed of light (almost). Nerve cells' outer lining consists of capsules of fatty material lined up alongside each other, with small gaps of exposed nerve cells in between them. These fatty capsules are known as the myelin sheath and the exposed areas are known as the nodes of Ranvier. With this set-up, the electrical impulse can jump along the nerve cell between nodes, covering a greater distance in a much shorter time. Omega-3 fatty acids are key to the development and maintenance of the myelin sheath, and just as essential for cognitive development.

Up to the age of two years old, the rate of lipid (fat) and protein accumulation in the brain is extremely high. Omega-3 isn't one single nutrient: it is actually a family of them. The ones most important to the growth and development of infants are EPA and DHA. These come exclusively from fish and seafood.

It is recommended that omega-3 fatty acids be supplemented by women planning to get pregnant, and during pregnancy, as many studies are beginning to show that sufficient levels in the mother will impact foetal neurological development.[1,2,3]

BEST SOURCES OF OMEGA-3
- Salmon
- Mackerel
- Herring
- Trout

The above are the two main nutrients that are essential and need attention, but this is against the backdrop of a wholesome, varied diet of fresh fruit, veg, meats, dairy, etc. to ensure a good cross-section of nutrients in a day and the development of a more adventurous habit. I recommend the work of Annabel Karmel, a specialist in this area with great ideas for weaning.

Nutrition during the early years and pre-teens

After the first year, an infant's appetite begins to decrease quite noticeably as their growth rate starts to reduce to about half of what it was. At this stage there can be notable changes in appetite almost from one day to the next. Some days they can have the appetite of a horse; the next day they barely want to touch a morsel. They are very well primed to listen to their body's appetite signals, which will vary during periods of rapid growth and slower growth. During this highly formative time there are some nutrients that require a special focus.

Protein

This stage of life is indeed one of very rapid growth that requires vast amounts of amino acids to build the myriad proteins needed to develop new tissues. Children in this age group, particularly in the age five to ten group, can be expected to gain around 30cm (12 inches) in height and 12kg (26½lb) in weight as they grow and develop. The recommended intake of protein for children in this age group is around 28g (1oz) per day. So, what does 28g (1oz) actually look like? The following charts give a few examples of the amounts of protein from common foods (there are lots of more expansive charts online, so do look them up if you need more information and make sure you consult a trustworthy source).

Food group	Food type	Protein in grams per 100g (3½oz)
Meat	Chicken breast (grilled without skin)	32.0
	Beef steak (lean grilled)	31.0
	Lamb chop (lean grilled)	29.2
	Pork chop (lean grilled)	31.6
Fish	Tuna (canned in brine)	23.5
	Mackerel (grilled)	20.8
	Salmon (grilled)	24.2
	Cod (grilled)	20.8
Seafood	Prawns (shrimp)	22.6
	Mussels	16.7
Eggs	Chicken eggs	12.5
Dairy	Whole milk	3.3
	Semi-skimmed (2%) milk	3.4
	Skimmed (skim) milk	3.4
	Cheddar cheese	25.4
	Half-fat cheddar	32.7
	Cottage cheese	12.6

Food group	Food type		Protein in grams per 100g (3½oz)
	Whole milk yogurt		5.7
	Low-fat yogurt (plain)		4.8
		Plant protein	
Pulses (legumes)	Red lentils		7.6
	Chickpeas (garbanzo beans)		8.4
Beans	Kidney beans		6.9
	Baked beans		5.2
	Tofu (soya bean steamed)		8.1
Grains	Wheat flour (brown)		12.6
	Bread (brown)		7.9
	Bread (white)		7.9
	Rice (easy-cook boiled)		2.6
	Porridge oats (oatmeal)		11.2
	Pasta (freshly cooked)		6.6
Nuts	Almonds		21.1
	Walnuts		14.7
	Hazelnuts		14.1

Protein-rich foods are abundant and diverse. By following a varied diet, including the foods listed previously (but not exhaustively), getting the recommended 28g (1oz) per day is easily attainable.

Calcium

As these years are the time of growth spurts, the skeleton is growing and forming at a rapid rate. Birth length doubles by the age of three to four and the femur and tibia of a three-year-old are about half of their eventual full adult length. It is a period of increased linear growth – new skeletal muscle and bone tissue. This is the time to make sure that there is an adequate supply of the building blocks needed to ensure this growth demand can be met. The current recommendations are that children between one and three years consume in the region of 700mg of calcium per day. This would work out at around three portions of dairy foods per day. But dairy isn't the only source of this vital mineral. The plant kingdom offers great sources, too.

BEST SOURCES OF CALCIUM
- Dairy products
- Fortified drinks and non-dairy 'milks'
- Tofu
- Broccoli
- Kale
- Beans and pulses (legumes)

Vitamin D

Vitamin D goes hand in hand with calcium, and its importance during such intense skeletal development is immense because vitamin D is needed to put calcium to use. Calcium is just one part of the skeletal health picture. I use the analogy of bricks on a building site. The bricks are the main structural material that walls are made of, but walls don't build themselves. You need a team of builders and specialists to take that structural material and expertly craft it into the end product – a building. It is the same with calcium. It IS the structural material of the skeleton, but it needs a team of other nutrients – vitamin D – to put it to use. Vitamin D takes calcium out of the blood to where it can be used.

We are in a time where vitamin D deficiency is beginning to appear again and rickets is making a return. This is a disease that all but vanished in Victorian times, but it has made a comeback. One hypothesis for this is the overuse of sunscreen. The primary source of vitamin D for humans is the conversion of cholesterol into vitamin D precursors when we are exposed to ultraviolet radiation (UV rays). Some have said that the big focus upon sunscreen use has been behind the sudden increase in this condition. Now, it is in no way my place to make any recommendation here. I am not a doctor or dermatologist. I am a nutritionist, so must stick to my remit, but this makes for food for thought.

Vitamin D is also believed to influence mood and immune function, and evidence is growing in that respect. We know, for example, that almost every cell in every tissue contains a vitamin D receptor, and that patients with noted vitamin D deficiency have lowered immune responses. Understanding of the exact mechanisms here is in its infancy, but we can see that vitamin D seems to have a regulatory role in key immune cell development.

BEST SOURCES OF VITAMIN D
- Full-fat dairy products
- Oily fish
- Eggs
- Offal

Omega-3 fatty acids

Just as in infancy, omega-3 fatty acids remain important at almost every stage of development, not to mention through into adult life. The brain and nervous system will be evolving at an astounding rate and require the right building blocks to ensure this development achieves its peak potential. New neuronal pathways will be developing as their learning goes through varying phases, and especially when they begin to talk and interact socially and go to school. These phases cause new neuronal growth and development in the brain, and a constant stream of omega-3 fatty acids supports this. Also, tissues are growing very quickly and new cells are being produced at lightning speed. Omega-3 fatty acids ensure the development of healthy cell membranes.

BEST SOURCES OF OMEGA-3
- Salmon
- Mackerel
- Herring
- Trout

Vitamin A

It is believed that one in ten children under five in the UK is deficient in vitamin A. This fat-soluble nutrient facilitates the functioning of the immune system, keeping the skin healthy and aiding night vision. Rely on food sources for vitamin A; it can be toxic if taken in supplements without professional advice.

BEST SOURCES OF VITAMIN A
- Full-fat dairy products
- Oily fish
- Orange fruit and veg (for the beta carotene form of vitamin A)

Nutrition from teens to twenties

Adolescence is certainly a tumultuous time. Changes are rife and can be aggressive at times. Puberty hits and can rock the boat in a hundred different ways. The development that occurs in puberty is what ultimately leads to final adult height, shape, body composition and physical and sexual function. This growth spurt doesn't create a drastic jump in nutritional needs in the same way as in early childhood, but there is still a slight increase in nutritional needs. At this stage, boys' and girls' requirements begin to differ. In boys, there is an increase in lean muscle tissue; in girls, a greater accumulation of adipose tissue – body fat. In both boys and girls, however, there is a rapid increase in bone density, so this formative stage creates specific nutritional requirements around that.

The recommendation is to follow the guidelines around protein, calcium and omega-3 set out in Nutrition During the Early Years and Pre-teens (see pages 12–17). Please visit that for greater detail.

Self-image, dieting and eating disorders

One thing that saddens me greatly, and something I can relate to in many ways as I had quite bad acne, is the potentially destructive nature of negative self-image in relation to our peers. At this stage of life we become far more conscious of ourselves: our bodies, faces and lives. All of it. It is a time of great vulnerability. This consciousness is amplified in the first instance by being surrounded by our peers every day at school. It is amplified further by the images of perfection portrayed by the media – super-slim, super-buff, smooth-skinned individuals paraded around in adverts on screen and in print.

The final factor that sends this up to level ten is social media. I am so glad that when I was at school, the internet didn't even exist (yep, I'm that old). Social media can become a personal hell for some and I have worked with teenagers that had been through unimaginable trauma because of it. It is a platform through which people are ultimately judged on such superficial attributes. I see it myself in the nutrition world especially, where six-pack-sporting 20-somethings are positioned as figureheads and spokespeople for nutrition when they have only done five minutes of study. It's a funny old world, driven by some very strange things.

With all of this in mind, it is no wonder that we consistently see alarming patterns of dieting and unhealthy relationships with food among teenagers in developed countries. A staggering 30% of teenage girls in the UK are on some diet or other. These are diets that are not developed under the guidance of a qualified practitioner to tackle serious weight problems or medical conditions – they are fad diets, diets filling the pages of magazines, diets that are developed as quick-fix miracles. This is a very worrying thing indeed.

The real concern is where these early unhealthy relationships with food can lead. Eating disorders are taking a dramatic upturn. Issues such as anorexia nervosa, bulimia nervosa and emotionally driven eating patterns are plaguing thousands now. You may think this is something that only girls suffer with; not at all. In the UK, 11% of those with an eating disorder are male. Whether you are a parent or a teenager reading this, having a greater insight into what these conditions are and their possible signs is an important thing. There are many eating disorders, from emotional eating to orthorexia (an obsession with eating only food that the sufferer perceives as healthy). The two most common ones, though, are anorexia nervosa and bulimia nervosa.

Anorexia nervosa

Anorexia nervosa is an illness where individuals purposely keep their body weight low. This is done by exerting extreme control through regimented eating patterns, refusal to eat, excessive exercising and even the use of laxatives. Anorexia can be an offshoot of body dysmorphia, whereby sufferers are convinced that they are overweight and see themselves as fat, no matter what their body weight is. When this condition arises in teenage girls, menstrual cycle-related issues may arise, like amenorrhea (when periods stop). There can also be a serious risk to skeletal health. The cycle disruptions can influence hormone levels, and the radically reduced nutritional intake can mean that important nutrients such as calcium and vitamin D are lacking during an important stage of bone density formation.

SIGNS TO LOOK OUT FOR
- Preoccupation with food, weight and body image
- Hiding eating patterns/food or lying about what they have eaten
- Avoidance of family meals or eating around others
- Irritability and moodiness
- Amenorrhea (when periods stop)

Bulimia nervosa

Bulimia nervosa is very closely related to anorexia in terms of the driving factors behind it: an intense fear of gaining weight or a very distorted body image. The difference in this condition is that there is a continual loop of binge eating followed by purging, which usually takes the form of self-induced vomiting. Many bulimia sufferers display a characteristic erosion of the teeth after a long period of the disorder due to the corrosive effects of stomach acid on the teeth from repeated vomiting.

SIGNS TO LOOK OUT FOR
- Disappearing soon after eating
- Mood swings and anxiety
- Amenorrhea (when periods stop)
- Patterns of weight gain and loss
- Depression and low self-esteem

General dietary patterns

General dietary patterns for adolescents still need to be
built around that ideal intake model – non-starchy vegetables,
complex carbohydrates and good-quality proteins. A focus
on getting as much wholefood into them as possible is the
order of the day. Minimize refined or overly processed foods
like ready meals, packaged snacks, etc.

Nutrition in the twenties to fifties

This big chunk of the lifespan is what I think of as the 'maintenance' era, the time where we need to do our utmost to maintain good health and healthy habits so that we make it through to the final chapter. However, this is often the time when our health becomes a lower priority. In early adulthood we are often highly social creatures who like to party and be out there in the world, hoovering up as many amazing formative experiences as we can, and rightfully so. In this hedonistic time of personal growth, search for identity and immersion in the world, we can often overlook the simple things like eating well and looking after our bodies.

The thirties and forties tend to be the career- and child-dominated years – the years where we find our feet in our careers and begin to excel. We often find ourselves in times of great stress, driven by deadlines, bills, commitments and, for many, family life, too.

The fifties are a time when we often truly see our successes come to fruition, still very much career focused. Many people experience changes of mind and heart in the fifties, and health suddenly becomes more important once again. Many report feeling the wear and tear beginning to show.

Watching the waistline

The twenties to fifties are a time when our waistlines can begin to go through something of a growth cycle, but not usually a planned one. Our energy needs don't change at all (apart from during pregnancy) from the ages of 20 to 50. However, with shifting life priorities and stresses can come poorer food choices (takeaways, ready meals, convenience foods, comfort eating, etc.) and, for many, a more sedentary lifestyle as work takes over our lives. In the UK and the US, around two-thirds of us are overweight, with around 25% falling into the obese category. Those are scary numbers.

Following these simple guidelines can in itself have a huge impact, as we are working directly with our physiology in a way that doesn't cause the metabolic chaos that is behind much of the weight gain we see in our population.

Protection and prevention

In my eyes, the key nutritional focus for this period of life is protecting ourselves against many of the degenerative conditions that healthcare systems in the developed world are swamped with and that can essentially be considered 'lifestyle' diseases. Heart disease, obesity, type 2 diabetes, cancers. They are on the rise at alarming rates and the healthcare system in the UK, for example, is set to burst. I'd love to say that there were real solid magic bullets that could save us from all these woes, but there aren't. There ARE, however, some simple eating patterns that can have profound effects.

Reduce refined carbohydrates

Refined carbohydrates (white bread, white rice, white pasta and simple sugars) can all send our blood sugar levels rising very quickly. So why is this a problem? Several damaging things can start to occur. When blood sugar rises, the body responds by releasing the hormone insulin. Insulin tells our bodies that glucose is available and opens doorways in the cell wall to allow glucose in. This glucose can then be turned into ATP (adenosine triphosphate), the energy source we run on. The problem is that our cells have a cut-off point; they can only allow so much sugar in at one sitting. They become full and then they shut the door.

When this happens, if blood sugar is still high, it has to come down. So what happens is that the excess sugar gets sent to the liver, where it is converted into a fat called triacylglycerol, otherwise known as triglycerides. These are a type of fat designed for storage. They are sent to the fat cells within our adipose tissue, i.e. the fat around the stomach, where they can be stored almost like an energy rainy-day fund. So, the first part of the story is that too much sugar that is elevated for too long can lead to abdominal weight gain. The second – and probably most dangerous – part of the story is that this fatty substance has to be transported to the fat cells via our circulatory system. As the triglycerides travel through our circulation, they are susceptible to oxidation, which can cause damage to the endothelium lining the inside of our blood vessels. This damage sets off a cascade of events that eventually leads to plaque formation – the key underlying element of heart disease.

Now just when you thought the picture couldn't get any worse, a third thing happens. If we continue to follow a diet that constantly raises blood sugar to such an excessive degree, in time the receptors that detect insulin signals start to become less sensitive to the signal that insulin is delivering. This is a state known as insulin resistance whereby the cells of the body do not receive the signals that insulin is sending out as effectively as it once did. This means that cells cannot react and take up available glucose as effectively as before. This, in turn, leads to elevated blood glucose, which goes on to exacerbate the problem. The next stage after that is type 2 diabetes.

The simplest way to avoid this whole ugly picture is to swap your everyday white carbs for the brown ones. Swap white rice for brown rice, white pasta for wholewheat pasta, etc. The brown or multigrain versions have a much higher fibre content, and because of this they take much longer to digest, liberating their sugars much more slowly. This causes a gentle drip-feeding of blood sugar instead of a complete carpet bombing.

Reduce vegetable oils

The second big thing we can do for long-term health and protection against disease is reduce our intake of vegetable oils. By this I mean oils like sunflower oil, or soya oil or corn oil. These oils are incredibly high in a type of fatty acid called omega-6. Now, the omega-6 fatty acids are vitally important to our health, but we only need them in minute amounts. When we take in more than we need, they get transformed into things called series 2 prostaglandins, which switch on and exacerbate inflammation. The inflammation I'm talking about isn't like a sudden acute inflammation where your ear swells up to twice its size, rather subclinical inflammation that can only be detected via something like a blood test. Chronic subclinical inflammation in tissues has been linked to many degenerative diseases such as heart disease and certain types of cancer.

Instead of using these oils, I recommend opting for a good-quality extra virgin olive oil, as this doesn't upset the inflammatory response at all.

Increase nutrient density

The final golden rule for everyday health throughout this part of life is to ensure maximum nutrient density every time you eat. This is really simple to achieve: try to ensure you have some fresh, minimally processed plant foods on your plate at every meal. This could be as simple as a good-quality side salad. It could mean snacking on fresh fruit between meals or making veg one of the major parts of your main course. Why does any of this matter? Well, this is where your micronutrition comes from. The micronutrients of the vitamins and minerals contain trace elements and phytoprotectants. Ensuring a micronutrient-dense diet helps to prevent any of the issues associated with nutritional deficiency. Adhering to these simple guidelines can stand you in great stead during this maintenance period.

Nutrition and ageing

Whether we like it or not, time takes its toll on our bodies...

Degenerative loss of skeletal muscle mass (sarcopenia)

Body composition can change in drastic ways as we age. One of the big changes is that we begin to lose muscle mass, known as muscle atrophy. This loss of muscle mass is increased in women after the menopause, and equal in both sexes at around the age of 80. The decline of muscle mass begins at about 30 years of age and occurs at a rate of around 5% per decade. After the age of 60, this rate of decline increases to around 10% per decade. As there is less metabolically active tissue, this decline in muscle mass also causes a decline in energy intake as requirements go down. Appetite and food intake can begin to decrease, which in turn affects intake of key micronutrients. It is common for intakes of vitamin D, magnesium, calcium and zinc to be low in the ageing population.

There are a few steps that can be taken to reduce the extent of this muscular mass decline, the biggest being resistance exercise such as lifting weights and using resistance machines. This, coupled with increased protein intake, can offer considerable protection against loss of muscle mass, and will also keep metabolism revved up and the appetite strong.

Reduced bone density

The density of the skeleton declines with age and there are a few factors to blame. The first factor is a decrease in the circulating levels of vitamin D. This can be caused by a reduction of vitamin D synthesis in the skin: the primary source of vitamin D for humans is the conversion of cholesterol into vitamin D precursors when the skin is exposed to ultraviolet radiation (UV rays), and the capacity to do this declines with age. Additionally, with age the amount we eat can reduce, and the micronutrient density of the diet declines. Supplementation with vitamin D, even as low as 200 IU a day, can prevent major complications. I, however, am in favour of intakes a bit higher than that level.

The second factor to affect bone density is calcium intake and utilization. As total food intake goes down, so does micronutrient intake, and levels of calcium in the diet begin to reduce lower. When this is coupled with vitamin D deficiency, you get a double whammy. Vitamin D actually takes calcium out of the bloodstream and sets it to work in the skeleton. If both of these nutrients are low, things can get serious. Ensuring an adequate intake of calcium-rich foods is essential.

One of the big age-related factors in bone density loss in women is the menopause. The drop in the hormone oestrogen negatively affects bone mineralization.

The final factor that negatively impacts bone density is lack of exercise. Physical activity is a fundamental pillar in maintaining bone density, so ensuring some degree of activity is of the utmost importance.

B12 deficiency

A deficiency in vitamin B12 is common in older adults for two reasons. The first – a recurrent theme here – is reduced food intake and variety. At this stage of life many factors influence food intake: financial strain, mobility issues, solitude. All of these things can influence food choices, and lack of dietary variety is common in the elderly.

The second reason is a drop in the levels of something called intrinsic factor (IF). This is a glycoprotein produced by cells in the stomach called parietal cells, and it plays a very important part in the absorption of vitamin B12. As we age, production of this important complex decreases, greatly hampering absorption. Note that B12 only exists in animal foods.

BEST SOURCES OF VITAMIN B12
- Red meats
- Offal
- Oily fish
- Eggs

B12 supplements are a definite consideration here (see page 220 for more information).

Reduced immune function

As life progresses there is a consistent, albeit slow, decline of immune tissues. Age can bring with it some reduction in the function of the different cells and responses within the immune system, much of which is related to an individual's nutritional status.

One of the most common deficiencies responsible for impaired immune function in the elderly is zinc deficiency, even though only very small amounts are needed. Zinc is used by our white blood cells to code genes that regulate the way in which these cells actually respond to pathogens they come into contact with. These genes determine the type of response, so any impairment can drastically alter immune response.

BEST SOURCES OF ZINC-RICH FOODS
- Prawns (shrimp)
- Pumpkin seeds
- Walnuts

Cognitive decline

One aspect of ageing is cognitive decline, which can take devastating turns. Cognitive decline is inevitable to some degree, but there have been significant links made between nutrition and the rate and extent to which this can happen.

B vitamins are one group of nutrients that have been widely studied in this context – B6 and B12 in particular. This is because of their ability to break down a substance called homocysteine. This is an amino acid that occurs naturally in the body during a process called methylation. Its metabolism and breakdown are reliant on cofactors that are formed from B6 and B12. If these nutrients are lacking, then levels of homocysteine can rise, and elevated levels of it have been associated with increased cardiovascular disease risk, and cognitive decline. Many trials have shown that B vitamin supplementation can slow cognitive decline. The University of Oxford's VITACOG Study (2010) assessed 266 people over the age of 70 with diagnosed mild cognitive impairment. A daily combination of folic acid, B6 and B12 was associated with an average 30% reduction in homocysteine levels, which resulted in improvements in a range of mental tests including global cognition and episodic memory.[4]

Flavonoids are a group of phytochemicals that have also been associated with improved cognitive function, due to their impact on circulation. Flavonoids are compounds found in foods that give blue/purple colour pigments. Foods such as blueberries, blackberries, red wine, chocolate and green tea are all rich in them, and there are associations between high intakes of these and improved cardiovascular and cognitive health. Flavonoids affect the circulation by enhancing blood flow. They are taken up by the endothelial cells that make up the inner lining of our blood vessels, and when this occurs, the flavonoids appear to cause some type of alarm response within the cells, prompting them to secrete high levels of nitric oxide (which they secrete anyway). The nitric oxide moves from the endothelial cells out into the muscular walls of the blood vessels and causes the muscle fibres to relax. As the fibres relax, the vessels get wider. This lowers blood pressure and enhances circulation and blood flow. It is believed that this enhanced blood flow increases oxygen saturation in the brain.

BEST SOURCES OF FLAVONOIDS
- Blueberries
- Blackberries
- Red onions
- Red wine
- Very dark chocolate
- Green tea

Omega-3 fatty acids

The omega-3 fatty acids EPA and DHA are vitally important constituents in the brain and influence cognitive function in a number of ways. They are involved in keeping cell membranes healthy and fluid, especially a specialized type of membrane on nerve cells called the myelin sheath that is vital for relaying signals through the brain. They also regulate the function of receptors for different neurotransmitters that are also part of the signal relaying cycle. One key area is the impact that they have on inflammation. EPA and DHA are the building blocks of compounds that manage inflammation in the body, such as prostaglandins and resolvins. Inflammation is believed to be linked to many neurodegenerative processes. There is also some evidence to suggest that DHA, in particular, can improve areas of the brain affected by amyloid plaques in Alzheimer's. A great deal of epidemiological data (the study of disease patterns among populations) has shown an association between high omega-3 intakes through foods such as oily fish and decreased risk of cognitive decline. It must be noted, though, that epidemiological studies show association, not necessarily causation, but there is a great deal of plausibility behind how these fatty acids could offer protection.

BEST SOURCES OF OMEGA-3
- Salmon
- Mackerel
- Herring
- Trout

REFERENCES

1) Daniels JL, Longnecker MP, Rowland AS, Golding J, ALSPAC Study Team. 'Fish intake during pregnancy and early cognitive development of offspring.' *Epidemiology. 2004 Jul: 15(4): 394–402*

2) Helland IB, Smith L, Saarem K, Saugstad OD, Drevon CA. 'Maternal supplementation with very-long-chain n-3 fatty acids during pregnancy and lactation augments children's IQ at 4 years of age.' *Pediatrics. 2003 Jan; 111(1): electronic edition 39–44*

3) Larque E, Demmelmair H, Koletzko B. 'Perinatal supply and metabolism of long-chain polyunsaturated fatty acids: importance for the early development of the nervous system.' *Ann N Y Acad Sci. 2002 Jun; 967: 299–310*

4) de Jager CA, Oulhaj A, Jacoby R, Refsum H, Smith AD. 'Cognitive and clinical outcomes of homocysteine-lowering B-vitamin treatment in mild cognitive impairment: a randomized controlled trial.' *International Journal of Geriatric Psychiatry. 2012 July; 27 (6): 592–600*

A–Z of Common Ailments

There is really no getting around the fact that diet is a very powerful tool when it comes to our long-term health. Hopefully, this book makes it abundantly clear that our diet is a vital tool in disease prevention and is also essential for the proper growth and development of our bodies throughout the life span. I hope the conclusion that you draw from here is that diet acts as a potentially powerful intervention too. It has the power to become a therapeutic modality in its own right. In certain ailments, issues and health concerns, I absolutely believe that this is the case, and the evidence supports this. Then in other scenarios and with other health concerns, diet is completely irrelevant.

This chapter is an overview of the established information that we have on the role that nutrition can play in the treatment and/or management of some of the most common health concerns. If a common ailment is not on this list, it is simply likely that diet is irrelevant in its prevention or treatment.

ACID REFLUX

Acid reflux, more correctly called gastroesophageal reflux disease (GERD), is one of the most common gastrointestinal issues. While not serious in and of itself – more of an annoyance – long-term chronic reflux can give rise to a condition known as Barrett's oesophagus whereby the state of oesophageal tissue changes over time. This, in turn, can increase the risk of oesophageal cancer in some cases.

Acid reflux is experienced as a powerful burning sensation in the chest and throat. It is caused by the lower oesophageal sphincter not closing properly, and the highly acidic contents of the stomach leak up into an environment not built to cope with acid. Experiencing this now and again is pretty harmless, but if it becomes a regular occurrence, far more serious health problems can eventually arise, such as Barrett's oesophagus.

Nutritional Therapy for Acid Reflux

Eat little and often
Many patients report that eating smaller meals more frequently eases symptoms. The reason for this is that very large meals can stretch the stomach and put undue pressure on the lower oesophageal sphincter. It's the sheer volume of food in the stomach that can stretch the whole structure, distorting the sphincter and preventing it from closing properly.

Reduce fatty foods
Fatty foods such as heavy, oil-based dressings, dairy products and fatty meats have long been linked with exacerbating the symptoms of GERD. These fatty foods stimulate the secretion of higher levels of hydrochloric acid (HCL) in the stomach and slow down gastric emptying, keeping food in the stomach for longer.

Reduce alcohol

Sorry to be the bearer of bad tidings, but alcohol can notably weaken the lower oesophageal sphincter. This weakness means that the sphincter doesn't have sufficient muscle tone to close fully. However, this is a temporary state that can be improved by abstaining from drinking.

So, while you are suffering at least, try your best to keep alcohol intake at zero!

ACNE

Acne is an infection of the pilosebaceous unit – the area where the hair follicle and oil-producing gland meet in the skin. Oils in the skin become more viscous and can block the pore. Structural substances such as keratin get caught up in this viscous sebum and cause a plug to form that we call a blackhead. This blockage can trap bacteria that lives naturally on the skin's surface within the pore, which causes the immune system to instigate a response. The localized inflammatory response triggered in the early stages of this process is responsible for recruiting key cells of the immune system. They migrate to the area and begin to engulf and break down the bacteria. This causes pus to form and fill the pore area, resulting in the familiar whitehead spot and its associated swelling and pain.

Nutritional Therapy for Acne

Reduce inflammation with omega-3

Omega-3 fatty acids are metabolized to manufacture our body's own in-built anti-inflammatories – prostaglandins. Increasing our intake of omega-3 as much as possible, from either oily fish or supplements (nuts and seeds don't do the same job), increases the production of the prostaglandins that reduce inflammation. Supplement-wise, you need to aim for a dosage of around 750mg EPA (eicosapentaenoic acid) per capsule. EPA is the omega-3 fatty acid that feeds straight into the pathway that gives rise to the powerfully anti-inflammatory series 3 prostaglandins. Since the redness and pain associated with acne come from inflammation, reducing this will make acne flare-ups look less severe and feel less painful.

Fight infection with zinc

The mineral zinc is a powerful tool in supporting the immune system. It is used by white blood cells to control the way they respond to infection, making them far more effective infection-fighting machines.

Top Foods

Omega-3
Salmon
Mackerel
Herring
Fresh tuna

Zinc
Prawns (shrimp)
Scallops
Tuna
Pumpkin seeds
Almonds
Walnuts

ANXIETY

Anxiety is a condition that seems to be ever on the increase. In fact, according to NHS UK, it is estimated that around 4.7% of the UK population experience anxiety, and around 9.7% experience anxiety combined with depression.

This is really quite a shocking picture but, with the madness that is modern life, also unsurprising. Generalized anxiety disorder (GAD), while affecting 5% of the population, actually accounts for almost 30% of the mental health issues seen by GPs. It is a condition where, in most cases, the sufferer still feels relatively in control and is conscious of the problem, so taking themselves along to their GP is more common than would be the case with other, more serious mental health concerns.

Anxiety is normal and necessary. When we perceive a threat or a situation that is potentially harmful or problematic, the physiological workings of our body respond very quickly and go into 'fight or flight' mode. A small gland at the very base of our brain, the pituitary gland, is the first part of our body to get involved: when the signal of perceived threat comes from the brain, the pituitary springs into action and secretes a number of signalling hormones. These hormones fly through our bloodstream to the adrenal glands that sit above our kidneys. The adrenal glands pump out adrenaline, which makes the heart pump faster, our breathing quicker, our muscles to become tense and our minds to become focused on the potential hazard. This all happens at lightning speed, and our only perception of it is when we are right in the middle of it.

Nutritional Therapy for Anxiety

Maintain nerve cell health with omega-3 fatty acids
These fatty substances are vital for the maintenance of the myelin sheath, the fatty outer lining of our nerve cells,

which is essential for the proper transmission of information throughout the nervous system. Fatty acids are vital for regulating the function of neurotransmitter receptors – molecules that receive the signal delivered by neurotransmitters, enabling neurotransmission (the transmission of nerve impulses). Many studies (such as Kiecolt-Glaser JK, Belury MA, Andridge R, Malarkey WB, Glaser R. 'Omega-3 supplementation lowers inflammation and anxiety in medical students: a randomized controlled trial.' *Brain Behav Immun.* 2011 Nov; , 25(8): 1725–1734) have shown a reduction in anxiety with increased omega-3 intake, and it is believed that its role in maintaining this system is what offers the benefit.

Calm things down with magnesium

This vital mineral is involved in over 1,000 chemical reactions in the body. It can make us feel very relaxed, as it is involved in physically relaxing muscle. Calcium causes muscle fibres to contract, whereas magnesium induces them to relax. Increased magnesium can help us to feel physically less tense overall, thus reducing the severity of panic attacks when they occur. Magnesium also causes us to secrete higher levels of the neurotransmitter GABA (gamma-aminobutyric acid). This is the primary inhibitory neurotransmitter, meaning it calms down the central nervous system.

Follow a low-GI diet to stop the rollercoaster

A diet high in simple sugars and quick-release carbohydrates such as white bread, white rice, white pasta, etc. can cause blood sugar levels to peak and then crash. This rollercoaster pattern can result in fluctuations of mood – feeling full of energy, then crashing and feeling tired. That is to anxiety attacks what petrol is to a fire, so keeping blood sugar stable is vital for helping regulate our mood. Swap your staple white carbohydrates for the brown and multigrain varieties.

Reduce their total portion size and combine them with good-quality protein to create a meal that takes longer to digest and, in turn, releases its energy slowly and evenly.

Top Foods

Omega-3	Magnesium	Low-GI carbohydrates
Salmon	Kale	Brown rice
Mackerel	Cavolo nero	Pearl barley
Herring	Savoy cabbage	Quinoa
Fresh tuna	Broccoli	Bulgur wheat
	Pumpkin seeds	
	Almonds	

ARTHRITIS

Arthritis is a very common phenomenon with, according
to NHS UK, over ten million people in the UK affected by it.
It affects all ages, not just the elderly, including young children.
There are many types of arthritis, the most common of which
are osteoarthritis and rheumatoid.

Osteoarthritis

This is the type of arthritis that basically could be described as
normal wear and tear of the joints. It could be due to advancing
age or, as in my case (I have it in the ankle – it isn't fun), from
injury. In normal, age-related wear and tear, cartilage – the
tough, flexible tissue that cushions our bones and is used to
being broken down and built back up again – becomes less able
to replenish itself. In time, areas of the underlying bones become
exposed and bony surfaces can begin to rub together, leading to
further destruction of the joint, stiffness and pain. Surrounding
tissues can become inflamed and painful, too.

Rheumatoid Arthritis

Rheumatoid arthritis is a completely different ball game. It is
still a degradation of the tissues within the joint with pain and
inflammation, but differs from osteoarthritis in that it is caused
by the immune system, which for unknown reasons is attacking
the tissues in the joint, causing damage, inflammation, pain
and even deformity. There have in recent times been strong
links found between bacterial infections and the instigation
of rheumatoid arthritis. Then, other cases seem to appear
almost at random. Whatever has been the trigger, there is
an over sensitization of the immune system at play that starts
to attack and degrade synovial tissues.

Nutritional Therapy for Arthritis

While the two most common forms of arthritis have varying causes, they share similar symptoms, and it is at this level that nutrition may offer some relevance.

Reduce inflammation with omega-3

Omega-3 fatty acids are certainly the most potent nutritional intervention for inflammatory issues. This is because they are converted into our body's own in-built anti-inflammatory compounds. This doesn't get rid of the problem at all, but does at least offer some relief from symptoms by easing the pain and stiffness that arises from the inflammation. There have been many trials to date focused on both rheumatoid and osteoarthritis that have shown reduction in pain and stiffness with increased omega-3 intake.

Top Foods

Omega-3
Salmon
Mackerel
Herring
Fresh tuna

ASTHMA

Asthma is a common condition that is part of the atopic triad of asthma, eczema and hay fever. These three conditions very often run in families and all arise from what is known as a type II hypersensitivity reaction. This is where the immune system has become highly sensitized to a specific stimulus. So, in hay fever it is pollen; in asthma it can be dust mites, certain foods or other allergens; and in eczema the culprits include certain wash products, metals, disinfectants or even the juice from fresh fruit and veg coming into contact with the skin. Asthma, eczema and hay fever are essentially the same condition manifested in different tissues. They are all type II hypersensitivity reactions, but triggered by different allergens in different tissues. The response is the same – it's just what triggers it and where that varies.

In asthma the response is localized to the bronchioles, which are the tiny passageways in the lungs. When the immune system is exposed to the right stimuli, a substance called histamine is released by a type of white blood cell called a mast cell. You may be familiar with antihistamine tablets if you are a hay fever sufferer. Well, histamine produces a localized inflammatory response that, in the case of asthma, causes breathing difficulties.

Nutritional Therapy for Asthma

Eat quercetin-rich foods

Quercetin is a flavonoid that can deliver an antihistamine effect by preventing a process known as mast cell degranulation. The mast cells contain granules filled with histamine, and when they get the relevant signal from the immune system, they release their histamine content so as to create a localized inflammation. This is done to help the immune system in normal circumstances, but in type II hypersensitivity reactions, it happens in an exaggerated manner to everyday things that are hard to avoid, so reducing the levels of histamine can be favourable. Foods such as red onions and red peppers (bell) are great sources of quertecin, or supplements can be considered.

Reduce inflammation with omega-3

As you will see consistently throughout this book, omega-3 fatty acids give us the building blocks our body needs to manufacture its own in-built anti-inflammatory substances – the prostaglandins. As asthma is inflammation, anything you can do to reduce this inflammation will help ease symptoms. Oily fish like salmon, mackerel, herrings, etc. are the best sources.

Increase vitamin C

Like quercetin, vitamin C can interact with mast cells in a way that also reduces degranulation and histamine release. Remember, the mast cells are the ones that contain vesicles (a type of sac) of histamine, and when combined with an allergen will release histamine into the local environment. This triggers localized inflammatory symptoms, such as red itchy eyes, blocked upper respiratory and nasal passages, etc. Reducing this series of events is key to managing symptoms.

Top Foods

Quercetin-rich foods	Omega-3	Vitamin C
Red onions	Salmon	Citrus fruits
Red (bell) peppers	Mackerel	Peppers (bell)
Red wine	Herring	Spinach
Green tea	Fresh tuna	Broccoli
	Anchovies	

BLOATING

Bloating is one of the most common digestive complaints presented to doctors, dietitians and nutritionists. It is really just a symptom, and one that is often an indication that other aspects of digestion are not happy.

Bloating can be caused by constipation and poor gut motility (the transit of its contents), low stomach acids or digestive enzymes and problems with gut flora, and can be a sign of intolerance to certain foods. With all of this in mind, managing bloating can often be a case of real detective work to try and get to the bottom of what is behind it. While that detective work is going on, there are a few nutritional strategies that you can employ to reduce the symptoms.

Nutritional Therapy for Bloating

Nurture gut flora

Our gut flora is the vast colony of bacteria that lives in our digestive system. There are trillions of these bacteria. They are responsible for so many aspects of our digestion, from physically breaking down compounds from our foods through to regulating how the digestive system functions and takes care of itself. Slight disruptions to this population can cause chaos. Certain substances from our foods require these bacteria to break them down. If there are insufficient numbers or too many of the wrong type, then this process can cause the production of large amounts of gas – which leads to bloating.

There are two courses of action to nurture our gut flora: one, eating *prebiotic* foods that feed the bacteria and allow them to grow and flourish; two, topping up bacteria numbers with *probiotic* supplements.

Drink more water

Simple to do, yet so often not done. Drink enough water.
Water causes the fibre in the food we eat to swell up to many
times its own size. When this happens, stretch receptors within
the gut wall are stimulated. This, in turn, stimulates peristalsis –
the rhythmical contraction of the gut wall that keeps everything
moving along. Constipation and poor gut motility are two of
the major causes of bloating. Keep 'regular' and it will make
the world of difference.

Ease symptoms with carminatives

There are some herbs that are commonly available in teas that
can break down and dispel gas. In old herbal terminology, these
were called carminatives. Great examples include peppermint,
chamomile, caraway and aniseed. Brewed into teas, these are
great sipped throughout the day to ease symptoms.

Top Foods

Prebiotic foods	Carminatives
Jerusalem artichokes (sunchokes)	Peppermint
Onions	Caraway
Garlic	Chamomile
Leeks	Aniseed
Sweet potatoes	

BRITTLE NAILS

Brittle nails are a very common cosmetic complaint. While it isn't unusual for these structures to split and break from time to time as they take a fair amount of physical trauma in our day-to-day life, especially in those that have very manual jobs, if nails split excessively or do so when not in the presence of physical trauma, then there may be some weakness present and nutrition can influence this.

The nails and hair are both made of the same material – a substance called keratin, which is a tough protein. Brittle nails can sometimes be determined as hard brittle and soft brittle. Hard brittle is usually caused by too little moisture in the nail, often from over-washing of the hands. Soft brittle nails, on the other hand, are usually associated with excess moisture, for example from prolonged exposure to some detergents.

However, there are some situations that can cause brittle nails that nutrition can influence. These are iron deficiency and poor protein digestion.

Nutritional Therapy for Brittle Nails

Increase iron intake

A very common cause of brittle nails, in women especially, is a low level of iron. This can affect many tissues, and nail disruptions are usually a very late sign of being low in iron and will soon progress into a condition known as koilonychia or spoon-shaped nails. Women display this more often due to the loss of iron during menstruation. To top levels up, you can approach it in two ways, the first being with food. Dark green leafy vegetables and some dried fruits (such as dried dates and semi-dried figs and apricots) can deliver good levels of a type of iron called non-haem iron. This isn't always that well absorbed, so a good tip is to have some vitamin C with it like a lemon juice-based dressing, or a glass of fresh orange juice, for example. Then there are foods like red meat that will deliver a good dose of haem iron.

The second next way to top up iron, particular during and just after menstruation, is via a supplement. Be careful, though, as the cheaper forms of iron, such as ferrous sulphate, can wreak havoc with the digestive system, causing constipation. Opt instead for a form known as 'gentle iron', aka iron bisglycinate.

Improve protein intake and protein digestion

Improving protein intake and digestion is a less common cause of brittle nails, but certainly won't go amiss in terms of making nails stronger and looking better overall. To improve protein intake, aim to get a good source of protein into each of your meals. This can be plant sources like tofu and tempeh, or indeed animal sources such as meat and fish. These foods will help to strengthen the keratin and give the nails a better, smoother and stronger appearance.

Improving protein digestion is the second part of the equation for some. The most suitable way to do this is to take a good-quality digestive enzyme supplement at the beginning of each meal to ensure effective digestion of all the additional protein foods you are consuming. It just helps to break it down into its component amino acids more efficiently.

COLD SORES

Cold sores are one of those non-serious but very unsightly and annoying afflictions that plagues millions of us. They arise following infection with the herpes simplex virus. Once we are exposed to this, we have it for life. Most of the time it is dormant, but if the immune system becomes weakened for whatever reason, it can trigger a cold sore attack.

Nutritional Therapy for Cold Sores

Support the immune system with zinc

One of the best ways to keep cold sores at bay is to support the immune system. Remember, once you have been exposed to the virus, there is no going back, so your best bet is to keep the immune system strong. Focus on extra zinc in the diet. Zinc is used by our white blood cells, the army of the immune system, to manufacture genes that regulate how effectively the immune system responds to pathogens and infected cells and tissues.

Tackle stress with B vitamins

Reducing the impact of stress can also help here, as prolonged stress can really influence the strength and effectiveness of the immune system. One of the key groups of nutrients to reduce the physiological impact of stress is the B vitamin group. These vitamins help to support the nervous system and reduce burn-out, which, in turn, can help prevent the immune system becoming ineffective.

Reduce inflammation with omega-3

I want to drive home how important these substances are for managing any kind of issue that involves inflammation. Extra omega-3 fatty acids from oily fish can help to ease some of the inflammation during a flare-up.

Top Foods

Zinc

Oysters

Prawns (shrimp)

Scallops

Walnuts

Pumpkin seeds

Sunflower seeds

Whole grains

Omega-3

Salmon

Mackerel

Herring

Fresh tuna

COLDS AND FLU

There is no cure as such, but we can support our bodies in a way that means our natural defences against colds and flu are greatly enhanced. Cold and flu viruses attack the upper respiratory tract, and this recruits the immune system to respond, causing inflammation in all of these upper respiratory tissues, which is what gives us the symptoms we are so familiar with.

Nutritional Therapy for Colds and Flu

Increase your intake of zinc

Zinc is the ONLY nutrient that has had consistent success in clinical trials against the common cold. Vitamin C has been notoriously unreliable in trials, yet is the nutrient that people still reach for when a cold comes knocking. Zinc is vital, as it is used by our white blood cells, the army of the immune system, to code genes that regulate the way in which they respond to pathogens. These genes control the types of responses that they deliver and how effectively they deliver them.

Reduce inflammation with omega-3

About 90% of the symptoms we experience during a cold are down to inflammation within the respiratory tract. Omega-3 fatty acids provide us with the building blocks for our body to make its own in-built anti-inflammatory compounds. By increasing our intake of omega-3, namely the varieties EPA and DHA that we find in oily fish, we can help to minimize inflammation.

CONSTIPATION

Constipation is one of the biggest scourges in the UK. According to NHS statistics, an estimated whopping 6.5 million people suffer with it at one point or another in their lives.

There are so many factors that can aggravate constipation, from taking iron supplements and medications through to the more obvious one of diet. Processed foods devoid of anything nutritious dominate so many of our diets in modern times, and addressing this is one of the key areas to start with.

Nutritional Therapy for Constipation

Up your fibre intake

This is probably the most important step towards managing constipation. Dietary fibre takes on many times its own weight in water and swells up significantly. When it swells up, it stretches the walls of the gut. This then activates stretch receptors within the gut wall, in turn stimulating peristalsis, the well-orchestrated rhythmical contraction process that moves our gut contents along and ensures that we stay 'regular'.

Low-fibre diets built around refined carbohydrates like white bread, white rice, processed foods, etc. have such a low fibre content that they greatly inhibit peristalsis and smooth movement of gut contents. Avoiding these and switching over to the high-fibre alternatives is the order of the day.

Drink more water. This simple suggestion is really to make that the increased fibre intake does what it is meant to do: swell up to stretch the gut wall and activate stretch receptors. BUT, you have to drink enough in the first place in order to allow this to happen. So aim for eight to ten glasses a day.

Top Foods

Oats

Beans and pulses (legumes)

Green leafy vegetables

Brown rice

Wholemeal breads

CYSTITIS

Cystitis is a very common, irritating but harmless urinary tract infection caused by *E. coli*. This is a bacteria that naturally lives in specific areas of the urinary tract as well as some parts of the digestive system, where it wouldn't normally cause any kind of infection or problem. However, if it gets the opportunity to travel to and proliferate in regions of the urinary tract where it wouldn't normally be present (e.g. the bladder), then infection can occur. At this point the immune system gets involved, and consequently the walls of the urinary tract become inflamed and discomfort sets in.

Nutritional Therapy for Cystitis

Opt for cranberries for prevention

Cranberries have long been used as a remedy against cystitis. This traditional treatment does have validity thanks to a group of colour pigment compounds called anthocyanins. These seem to have the ability to pull *E. coli* from the walls of the urinary tract, or at least prevent them from binding in the first place. However, many trials have shown that it makes a better deterrent than cure.

DEPRESSION

Just 15–20 years ago, depression was far less an accepted long-term medical condition, but with advances in research a nd campaigning from sufferers and support organizations, the recognition of this condition has greatly improved. In the UK, it is estimated that one in four women and one in ten men will, at some point in their lives, experience an episode of depression severe enough to warrant treatment. Most of these cases are in the mild to moderate category, and most will be treated in primary care. Women seem to be at higher risk of depressive disorders and associated morbidity. This is thought to be as a result of a combination of factors that commonly interact – biological, psychological and sociocultural. Women are, of course, also open to depression during and after pregnancy.

Nutritional Therapy for Depression

Enhance receptor function with omega-3

Neurotransmitter receptors are molecules that receive the signal delivered by neurotransmitters. These are chemicals that allow the messages sent along nerves in the form of an electric impulse to jump the gap between nerve cells. Neurotransmitters such as serotonin are associated with elevated mood. However, these chemical messengers need to be detected by receptors so that they can deliver their messages. If the receptors are not working well, the neurotransmitter's message will not be heard as clearly. Omega-3 fatty acids are vital for regulating the health and function of neurotransmitter receptors.

Omega-3 fatty acids also regulate the health of the nerve cell membrane, especially in areas at the nerve endings opposite neurotransmitter receptors. This is the area of the opposing nerve that releases neurotransmitters into the synaptic space (gap between neurons). The fatty acids ensure effective release.

Stock up on B vitamins

The B vitamins are a mutually dependent group of nutrients that play a vital role in neurological health. Vitamin B6, for example, regulates the manufacture of myelin – the fatty outer lining of nerve cells. It is also involved in the conversion of the amino acid tryptophan into the neurotransmitter serotonin. Tryptophan is important for development and growth. Also known as B9, folic acid has major links to depression when levels are low. It is involved in the manufacture of neurotransmitters, too.

The B vitamins are also involved in turning food into energy, and if your energy levels plummet, your mood quickly follows.

I highly recommend that you do not supplement with individual B vitamins, as people often do, but instead opt for foods that are naturally rich in a wide variety of them.

Up your serotonin with tryptophan-rich foods

Tryptophan is an amino acid (protein-building block) that gets converted into the feel-good neurotransmitter serotonin. It crosses the blood–brain barrier where it goes through several biochemical pathways to become serotonin. A tryptophan-rich snack before bed can be helpful for sleep. One tip is to make sure that you have it together with a carb-rich food; you need a slight insulin rise to drive the tryptophan where it needs to go.

Top Foods

Omega-3	B vitamins	Tryptophan
Salmon	Brown rice	Turkey
Fresh tuna	Barley	Bananas
Mackerel	Oats	Eggs
Herring	Quinoa	Tofu
	Multigrain breads	Salmon
	Yeast extract	

DERMATITIS

Dermatitis is an inflammation of the skin that can lead to damage of the upper layers of the skin. Eczema also does this, but it is known as 'atopic dermatitis' and has a slightly different cause, so has its own entry in this section of the book (see page 64).

Like eczema, contact dermatitis occurs when the skin comes into contact with an irritant of some kind. This is often a cleaning substance, detergent, cosmetic, etc. When this contact is made, it can trigger an immune response that subsequently causes aggressive inflammation within the upper layers of the skin. This manifests in an initial raised redness and itching, which is then followed by a rapid die-off of skin cells that results in a dry, flakiness of the skin.

Nutritional Therapy for Dermatitis

Increase omega-3 to reduce inflammation

You will see these vital fatty substances mentioned time and time again throughout this book when we discuss any issue that features inflammation as a part of it. Quite simply, there is nothing else from a nutritional perspective that can impact and reduce inflammation to the extent that omega-3 fatty acids can. This is because the long-chain varieties, EPA and DHA found in oily fish and in supplements, are the metabolic building blocks that our body uses to manufacture its own in-built anti-inflammatory substances called prostaglandins.

Get extra vitamin E

As this important, fat-soluble antioxidant can help the skin to retain more moisture, it can reduce the severity of dryness and flakiness that arise following the initial contact inflammation.

Keep a symptom diary

Okay, so this isn't a nutritional intervention, but this is one of the first strategies I would employ with my patients in clinic. This involves keeping a daily record of both your symptoms and your daily habits such as foods eaten, where you went, what you did, any substances you may have handled, etc. In time, this can identify what the causative factor(s) may be. Ultimately, stopping this type of dermatitis really comes down to identifying the aggravating factor(s) and avoiding it/them.

Top Foods

Omega-3	Vitamin E
Salmon	Avocado
Mackerel	Walnuts
Herring	Pumpkin seeds
Pollock	Sunflower seeds
Fresh tuna	

DIABETES (TYPE 2)

Diabetes affects over 2.8 million people in the UK. Up to 90% of these sufferers are affected by type 2 diabetes, according to Diabetes UK. It is sometimes called late-onset diabetes because it tends to develop later in life. Alarmingly, though, there are younger and younger patients presenting with the condition. It occurs when our body's sugar management system malfunctions. It begins with our cells becoming less sensitive to insulin. If our diets are composed in such a way that our blood sugar is constantly high, we end up secreting more and more insulin – the hormone that tells cells to take up glucose. At first this isn't such a huge problem and our cells respond accordingly. After a while, though, the insulin receptors on our cells begin to suspect that something is up and start paying less attention to insulin. This will continue to develop and get worse, and blood sugar control will begin to fail. When blood sugar is consistently high, many structures can become damaged, including the beta cells in the pancreas that secrete insulin. When that happens, we become diabetic.

The good news is that in many cases, and providing that there aren't severe secondary complications, type 2 diabetes can be hugely improved and sometimes turned around through diet.

Nutritional Therapy for Diabetes (Type 2)

Follow a low-GI diet

This means avoiding foods that will raise your blood sugar too high too quickly. Some of these foods are obvious, like chocolate and fizzy drinks. Others, however, are less so.

The simplest way to get on the right track is to avoid all of the white starchy staples – white bread, white rice, white pasta. Instead, opt for the wholemeal or multigrain versions, swapping white rice for brown, white pasta for wholewheat, etc.

These have a much higher fibre content and so take much longer to digest. Because they take longer to digest, they liberate their sugars far more slowly, which, in turn, drip-feeds your blood sugar rather than carpet-bombing it.

The next way to lower the glycaemic index of the diet is to make sure that there is protein with every meal. Look at your plate and think, 'Where is my protein here?' Add the protein to your low-glycaemic carbohydrates. Think chicken with brown rice and greens, wholewheat pasta with tuna, spinach and red onions, etc.

By following such a diet, you will be keeping your blood sugar consistently within manageable levels. This means more insulin is secreted. Over time, if things haven't got too bad, your body's insulin receptors can once again become more receptive to insulin signalling.

Top Foods

Grains	Pulses (legumes)	Proteins
Brown rice	Chickpeas	Salmon
Barley	(garbanzo beans)	Mackerel
Quinoa	Adzuki beans	Herring
Millet	Butter (lima) beans	Chicken
Buckwheat	Lentils	

DIARRHOEA

Diarrhoea is, for the most part, the body's response to some type of environmental influence that is causing distress or damage to the local environment, or has the potential to cause infection. The body responds with an exaggerated peristalsis. This is the natural rhythmical contraction of the gut wall that moves gut contents along to their final destination. The exaggerated peristalsis causes very forceful, frequent contractions that expel gut contents rapidly and faster than normal. During the usual passage of gut contents throughout the digestive system, from the small intestine onwards, water is absorbed from the intestine into the body gradually so that when the gut contents finally arrive in the bowel as a stool, it has shape and form to it. When exaggerated peristalsis kicks in, the gut contents can be expelled before much of the water has been absorbed, hence the watery, unformed stool that is produced.

Other causes of diarrhoea will be covered on the entry about irritable bowel syndrome (IBS; see page 89), but include certain dietary components drawing water into the gut, which creates a watery, unformed stool and urgency to defecate.

Nutritional Therapy for Diarrhoea

Replace lost electrolytes

One of the big issues from a nutritional perspective is that attacks of diarrhoea can cause a rapid loss of electrolytes. These are minerals such as sodium, potassium, calcium and magnesium that have literally thousands of roles to play in the body, from communication across all cell membranes to regulating neurological function and maintaining hydration. They are vital substances that are rapidly lost. It is unlikely that you will have a huge appetite if you are in the midst of a full-blown diarrhoea attack, so one of the best ways to keep your electrolytes topped up is by making salty broths and soups. Choose things like miso soup or vegetable soups that make good use of green leafy vegetables and are seasoned with sea salt.

Stay hydrated

This is absolutely vital. You will be experiencing significant water loss during such attacks and can get rapidly dehydrated. Aim for 2–3 litres (3½–5¼ pints/4¼–6⅓ US pints) a day during such attacks.

Top up with probiotics

This is a bit of a scatter-gun approach, but with any kind of acute digestive episode, topping up with probiotics is a great idea. This is because these types of beneficial bacteria regulate many aspects of gut health, from gut motility (movement to propel its contents) to even managing local inflammation. They can also help to fight bacterial infection by direct aggressive responses to the bacteria or by competing with them for space in the gut.

DIVERTICULITIS

Diverticula are bulging pockets that can form in the lower parts of the large intestine. Patients with diverticula are often unaware of their presence and they usually turn up in some other routine examination. Sometimes these pockets can become inflamed. This is when symptoms including abdominal pain, bloating, diarrhoea and constipation can arise. It is believed that lack of fibre is one of the causes of this condition, as low-fibre diets can cause increased pressure against the colon wall.

When these pouches appear, smaller particles of food can sometimes get caught up in them, which can stimulate or exacerbate flare-ups.

Nutritional Therapy for Diverticulitis

Increase your fibre intake
This is best achieved with fibre-dense vegetables including green leafy vegetables such as kale, and broccoli, as well as butternut squash and sweet potatoes. All these vegetables deliver large amounts of fibre but aren't made of small particles, unlike seeds and some grains that can get stuck in the diverticula and aggravate the condition.

Keep it light during flare-ups
During attacks, opt for soups and broths. Soups made from antioxidant-rich vegetables such as squash and carrots, and spices like ginger, will also offer a fair amount of anti-inflammatory support.

Top Foods

High-fibre foods

Green leafy vegetables

Broccoli

Brussels sprouts

Butternut squash

Sweet potatoes

Yams

Oats

Brown rice

ECZEMA

Eczema affects a whopping 15 million people in the UK alone, according to Allergy UK. Of course, this is to varying degrees. It involves a very exaggerated immunological response to certain stimuli that leads to inflammatory flare-ups within the skin. It is, in fact, the same condition as asthma and hay fever, which make up the atopic triad (see page 42).

Eczema is a type II hypersensitivity reaction where the immune system has become overly sensitized to a stimulus and reacts aggressively to it. When the immune system reacts to the stimulus, patches of the skin become inflamed. When the inflammation settles down, the damaged skin then begins to flake and die off.

Nutritional Therapy for Eczema

Keep a symptom diary

One of the first things I advise patients to do when they have eczema is to keep a symptom diary, a daily record of your symptoms and diet/lifestyle. After time, patterns may start to form. You may be able to see that certain foods, lifestyle choices, etc. aggravate the condition. Treating eczema is like detective work, as the stimuli can be so varied.

Reduce inflammation with omega-3

Omega-3 fatty acids provide the body with the metabolic building blocks that it uses to create its own in-built anti-inflammatory substances. These are called prostaglandins. Some prostaglandins switch inflammation on and make it worse, and others reduce it. The omega-3 fatty acids EPA and DHA are used to manufacture the prostaglandins that switch inflammation off and reduce it.

Eat more orange foods

Foods such as sweet potatoes, carrots and mangoes belong to a group of fat-soluble phytonutrients called carotenoids. The group includes beta carotene, which is responsible for their orange colour pigment. Carotenoids act as an antioxidant that can accumulate in the skin and offer localized anti-inflammatory activity.

Top Foods

Omega-3
Salmon
Mackerel
Herring
Fresh tuna

Carotenoid-rich foods
Sweet potatoes
Mangoes
Carrots
Spinach
Kale

ENDOMETRIOSIS

Endometriosis is a distressing condition that involves the growth of endometrial (uterine) tissue outside the womb. This tissue will be just as responsive to hormonal signalling as it would be within the womb. This causes pain and swelling, and can have some very serious implications for fertility, too.

Nutritional Therapy for Endometriosis

Consume phytoestrogen-rich foods

Phytoestrogens are a group of phytochemicals (plant-derived chemical compounds) with a chemical structure that is very similar to that of the hormone oestrogen – so similar that they can bind to oestrogen receptors. Even though they bind to the receptor, they don't actually deliver an oestrogenic response. However, they hog the receptor so that real oestrogen cannot get to it and therefore cannot deliver its effects.

Manage inflammation with omega-3

This recommendation is really a case of symptom management. Buffering inflammation will help to ease some of the painful swelling associated with endometriosis. Omega-3 fatty acids provide the body with the building blocks that it uses to make its own anti-inflammatory substances, so by increasing our intake, we ramp up the production of these inflammatory mediators.

Top Foods

Phytoestrogens	Omega-3 Fatty Acids
Miso	Salmon
Chickpeas	Mackerel
(garbanzo beans)	Herring

FATIGUE

Fatigue is quite normal. We all lead very busy lives and this can sometimes leave us feeling a little burnt out. However, if this carries on for too long, it can become difficult to pull ourselves through every single day. Thankfully, a few small dietary tweaks could start to perk you up a little.

Nutritional Therapy for Fatigue

Stick to a low-GI diet

One of the keys to maintaining our energy levels is keeping blood sugar stable. By following a low-GI diet, we consume foods that release their energy slowly. This gently drip-feeds ourblood sugar levels instead of carpet-bombing them.

So what does a low-GI diet look like? Basically, instead of your everyday white carbohydrate staples, swap over to multigrain or wholemeal varieties. Think brown rice instead of white; wholewheat pasta instead of white. These varieties have a much higher fibre content and take longer to digest. As they take longer to digest, they release their energy much more slowly. This keeps blood sugar levels nicely even, in turn ensuring stable energy levels.

Top up on B vitamins

These vitamins are essential for turning the glucose released from food into energy. When glucose enters the cells, it needs to be converted into adenosine triphospate (ATP) – to fuel our cells. The B vitamins are responsible for several stages of this process.

Stay hydrated

We know that even a slight drop in hydration can cause us to feel fatigued and mentally foggy with a general feeling of malaise, so aim to drink eight to ten glasses of water every day to avoid feeling dehydrated.

FLATULENCE

While it is perfectly normal to pass wind many times a day, often without even realizing it, it can sometimes become a real problem. In its milder forms, it can just be antisocial or embarrassing. However, as it gets more severe, it can be incredibly uncomfortable and cause immense social anxiety. In most cases, it is simply the food we eat that is causing the issue. Different foods can affect the bacteria in the lower gut in different ways, and all of us respond differently. But there are components in food that stimulate fermentation reactions by gut flora, and the by-product of this fermentation can be different types of gas. The only real way to tackle flatulence is mostly through trial and error. Certain foods may be more aggressive than others and it is an individual issue. So experimentation is the way forward, but there are some key things you could try.

Nutritional Therapy for Flatulence

Cook fruit and veg for longer

It is a good idea to eat well-cooked vegetables that aren't too fibrous. I am usually a fan of very lightly cooked vegetables in order to minimize nutrient loss, but sometimes these can leave certain sugars intact that cause excessive fermentation (see next recommendation). Stewed and well-softened veg and fruit can reduce the levels of these sugars. Also try adding probiotic yogurts, drinks and even supplements to support gut flora.

Reduce high-fibre legumes and vegetables

High-fibre foods such as beans, lentils, onions, Brussels sprouts and cauliflower all contain very large polysaccharides, which are complex sugars that don't get broken down higher up in the small intestine as the more simple carbohydrates do.

Instead, they are mostly broken down in the lower part of the large intestine by the bacteria that reside there. In most of us, this fermentation process is beneficial, as it encourages the growth of the bacterial colony and also causes the release of by-products, such as butyrate and propionate, that can benefit the health of the gut and regulate satiety. In others, excessive gas is produced as part of the fermentation process and this can cause bloating, cramps and flatulence.

Ease symptoms with carminatives

There are some herbs that are commonly available in teas that can break down and dispel gas. In old herbal terminology, these were called carminatives. Great examples include peppermint, chamomile, caraway and aniseed. Brewed into teas, these are great sipped throughout the day to ease symptoms.

HAEMORRHOIDS

Haemorrhoids are essentially varicose veins that form in the lower bowel and anus. They are distorted blood vessels that arise from pressure in the lower bowel, which mostly comes from constipation or persistant straining to defecate. The constant pressure causes distortion of the vessel walls and the valves in the vessels that usually assist in venous circulation. This distortion can make them protrude and also make them easily rupture and bleed.

Nutritional Therapy for Haemorrhoids

Increase fibre intake

This is one of the main keys. The average fibre intake in the UK is scarily low, as so many of us have become dependent on highly processed convenience foods. Upping fibre intake can take the pressure out of the bowel, it softens the stool. Fibre can take on many times its own weight in water, which makes the stool fluffier and places less pressure upon the bowel walls.

Increase water intake

So, fibre is the first part of the picture, but we have to take a second step in order to make the fibre do its job, and that is to drink enough water. Since fibre works by taking on many times its own weight in water, you need to make sure there is enough coming in. Aim for around 2 litres (3½ pints / 4¼ US pints) day as a good starting point, but make sure you stagger this intake across the day.

Top Foods

High-fibre foods

Oats

Brown rice

Lentils

Beans

Quinoa

Multigrain breads

Wholewheat pasta

HAIR LOSS

Hair loss can be extremely distressing, particularly when rapid. It can be related to several different situations, each of which features its own unique pattern and rate of loss. The first and most common is male pattern baldness (MPB), which can affect women, too. Male pattern baldness is so called because the male hormone testosterone is the driving force.

Women have testosterone, too, and this same issue can arise in women, particularly those with polycystic ovary syndrome (PCOS), who have higher than normal levels of testosterone for a woman. In male pattern baldness, testosterone in the hair follicle converts into dihydrotestosterone, which causes the follicle to shrink continually. Each new hair that forms is thinner than the one before until they eventually fade away to nothing.

The second potential cause of hair loss is alopecia. This is an autoimmune response where the body's immune system attacks the hair follicle. This causes inflammatory damage to the follicle leading to reduced functioning that gives rise to the distinctive bald patches.

The final potential cause is nutrient deficiency. Long-term deficiencies in iron, magnesium and vitamin B12 can all lead to hair loss.

Nutritional Therapy for Hair Loss

There is, in fact, very little that can be done from a nutritional point of view for hair loss other than addressing deficiencies, but some small influences are possible.

Increase zinc intake

Zinc does appear to be involved in reducing the conversion of testosterone into dihydrotestosterone. Over long periods, this may help to reduce the severity or slow the progression of male pattern baldness.

Address potential deficiencies

The big three nutrients – (iron, magnesium and vitamin B12) – that, when deficient, can be associated with hair loss are generally all found in a high-quality, high-strength multivitamin. Additional magnesium can be taken alongside at dosages of up to 400mg twice a day.

Top Foods

Prawns (shrimp)
Pumpkin seeds
Walnuts
Beef

HALITOSIS

Halitosis (bad breath) is most often caused by bacteria that reside on the gums, teeth and tongue. It can also be an indicator of digestive problems such as constipation or gastroenteritis, as well as a sign of gum disease. Obviously, certain foods and habits such as cigarette smoking can make matters worse.

Anyone with consistent halitosis should visit their dentist as the first port of call to rule out gum disease or any other localized issue. If this is an all-clear, then a digestive tune-up should be the next port of call.

Nutritional Therapy for Halitosis

Deodorizing your mouth

Include green tea and citrus fruit in your diet: green tea contains polyphenol compounds that are deodorizing, can reduce bacteria in the mouth and prevent tooth decay; citrus is deodorizing and stimulates saliva production. Saliva helps to thwart the growth of a lot of bacteria that can cause halitosis, and also keeps the internal surfaces of the mouth clean and hydrated.

Avoid sugary foods

Simple sugars such as those found in confectionery can ferment easily and that can create odour. Cutting down on these simple sugar-laden snacks can go a long way to reducing odour through fermentation.

Drink plenty of water

This will help any fibre in your diet to swell up, which stimulates peristalsis, the natural rhythmical contraction of the gut, and ensures that gut motility (movement of its contents) is maximized, reducing constipation.

Consider a course of probiotics

This will also help to enhance digestive transit and keep the gut healthy. Probiotics are the living bacteria that we find either in supplement form or in functional drinks and foods. These help to top up the levels of the good bacteria that already live in the gut. This bacterial colony helps to regulate many aspects of gut health, from gut transit through to maintaining the health of the tissues that make up the gut.

HANGOVER

We have all experienced these little devils from time to time, and they can vary from a mild annoyance to absolute carnage that can leave us bedridden for the day. Headaches, dizziness, sensitive to light, nausea, lack of concentration – we all know the feeling. Excessive alcohol can make the blood vessels swell, causing throbbing headaches and bloodshot eyes. There is inflammatory damage to the stomach and intestines, too, which causes the barrage of digestive maladies that accompany a hangover. Blood sugar levels can fluctuate like a rollercoaster, making you feel fatigued and even more light-headed.
Above all, it massively dehydrates you.

Nutritional Therapy for Hangovers

Grab some complex carbs and protein

The first thing to do is to get blood sugar in check by consuming some good-quality complex carbs and some high-quality protein. Imagine a breakfast like poached egg on multigrain toast: the complex carbs in multigrain toast take longer to digest, meaning that they drip-feed your blood sugar rather than carpet-bombing it with simple sugars such as those found in white bread. The latter approach will cause more problems later on, like making your energy plummet even further and making you even more light-headed and fatigued.

The protein from the egg will help to sustain blood sugar levels even further, but also supply amino acids that are used by the liver to make enzymes that break down and remove alcohol.

Top up your B vitamins

These water-soluble nutrients – so vital for energy production and mood stabilization – will be lost in abundance after drinking alcohol, as the increased urination quickly leaches them from the body. This can make you feel fatigued, have a mental fog and even feel more nervous and anxious.

Top up your electrolytes

Alcohol dehydrates you. Big time! This is caused by loss of electrolytes that maintain fluid balance. Minerals such as sodium, potassium and magnesium are all electrolytes and they will need replacing to get you hydrated again (not to mention the myriad other essential roles they have to play, such as regulating muscular contraction, nerve signalling and cellular communication). One of the easiest ways to do that is to add a good pinch of quality sea salt to a glass of water two to three times during the morning.

Get some extra vitamin C

A little bit of vitamin C wouldn't go a miss either. This is because it assists the liver in breaking down alcohol.

Top Foods

Complex carbohydrates	B vitamins	Vitamin C
Oats	Whole grains	Citrus fruits
Brown rice	Green leafy vegetables	Kiwi fruit
Quinoa	Eggs	Berries
Multigrain breads	Nuts and seeds	Peppers
Wholewheat pasta		(bell)
		Spinach

HEAVY, PAINFUL PERIODS

Periods can become overly heavy or excessively painful for many reasons. Conditions such as endometriosis (see page 66), fibroids and even thyroid problems can impact them. Then factors such as stress, environmental pollutants and the use of the contraceptive pill can all influence your menstrual cycle negatively, too.

Nutritional Therapy for Heavy, Painful Periods

Eat more oily fish
You will need to be well stocked up on those all-important omega-3 fatty acids. This is because they help to reduce inflammation by supplying the ingredients the body needs to manufacture its own in-built anti-inflammatory substances. This can help to ease some of the pain and excessive cramping.

Eat brightly coloured fruit and veg
Numerous studies have shown that a wide intake of brightly coloured fruits and vegetables is associated with reduced pain and severity of bleeding. The closer participants went to a plant-based diet, the better symptoms became. What hasn't been established is exactly why and how this is the case. It is likely due to the anti-inflammatory effects of the many antioxidant substances that are found in such foods. So, adopting a predominantly plant-based wholefood diet is a good way to ensure a steady supply of these key substances, as well as to crowd out a great deal of the pro-inflammatory substances that are found in some animal foods like red meat.

Eat iron-rich foods along with vitamin C
One thing that is obviously a concern when suffering from excessively heavy periods is iron loss through heavy bleeding.

This can lead to intense fatigue. Reaching for iron-rich foods is logical, but if you add a little vitamin C alongside these foods, iron absorption will be increased several times over.

Top Foods

Omega-3	Brightly coloured food examples	Iron-rich foods
Salmon	Red (bell) peppers	Red meat
Mackerel	Red cabbage	Poultry
Anchovies	Purple sweet potatoes	Dark green leafy
Pollock	Squash	vegetables
		Dried apricots

HIGH BLOOD PRESSURE

High blood pressure (BP), or hypertension, is one of the biggest risk factors for heart disease. Blood pressure is basically the pressure that is exerted against the wall of our blood vessels. Blood vessels expand and contract almost consistently to manage the pressure within the vessels and ensure circulation to all parts of our body. Age, lifestyle and activity levels can all have an influence upon how flexible our blood vessels are. If they lose flexibility and are combined with factors such as high sodium or high omega-6 diets, the pressure against the vessel wall increases, as does the risk of vascular injury. Also, if there are already areas of damage within the wall of the vessel, then increased pressure within that vessel could increase the likelihood of it rupturing, which will then lead to a blood clot that can potentially dislodge and travel through the circulatory system, eventually blocking off areas of tissue. That is what occurs in heart attacks and strokes.

With this in mind, keeping blood pressure under control is absolutely vital to our long-term health, and diet and lifestyle are huge determinants of this.

Nutritional Therapy for High Blood Pressure

Reduce sodium

You may well have heard the advice for years to reduce salt intake. That is only part of the picture. We need salts – they are important for almost every aspect of cellular health. Completely cutting out salt will result in a pretty rapid death, so we need to be a little clearer as to what the advice actually should be. What we need to do is reduce excess *sodium*.

In our modern diet, sodium tends to come from table salt. This nasty, stock- cupboard staple is pure sodium chloride. Sodium in excess can have two negative influences upon our blood pressure. Firstly, sodium slows down the movement of fluid through the filtration mechanism of the kidneys. This means that our body actually holds on to water for longer. Holding on to excess water means that the watery portion of our blood, otherwise known as plasma, increases in volume. As this volume increases, then simple physics kicks in: the volume within a vessel increases, therefore the pressure exerted against it will increase too.

The other way that sodium negatively influences our blood pressure is that it is vasoconstrictive, i.e. it causes contraction of the smooth muscle within the vessel wall, raising blood pressure.

Increase purple foods

Okay, this may sound a little odd, but hear me out. Purple foods such as blueberries, blackberries, red wine, etc. are all very rich in a group of compounds called flavonoids. These substances have been widely studied, particularly here in the UK, under Professor Jeremy Spencer at the University of Reading.

What we understand about flavonoids is that they are rapidly taken up by endothelial cells. The endothelium is the skin that makes up the inner lining of blood vessels. When endothelial cells take up flavonoids, the flavonoids trigger an alarm response within the endothelial cell. This causes the cell to secrete large amounts of a substance called nitric oxide. Nitric oxide then moves out into the smooth muscle that makes up the vessel wall and causes the muscle fibres to relax. As these fibres relax, the vessel dilates and the pressure within it drops.

Top Foods

Flavonoid-rich foods

Dark chocolate

Blueberries

Blackberries

Red onions

Red wine

Green tea

HIGH CHOLESTEROL

Cholesterol is vital as the building block in the manufacture of many hormones. It is also an important part of cell membranes as well as the precursor to vitamin D, so it's fair to say that it is pretty important stuff. The fact that large amounts are made in the liver every single day should be a good indicator of this.

Now, you may have heard of 'good cholesterol' and 'bad cholesterol' or words to that effect. There is no such difference. Cholesterol is cholesterol – there is only one type. What people mean are low-density lipoprotein (LDL) and high-density lipoprotein (HDL) cholesterol. These are basically transport mechanisms to carry cholesterol around the body. You could liken them to bus routes: one bus is going out of town; another is coming into town. Because LDL is carrying cholesterol away from the liver out into the body, it is somehow viewed as being bad. And because HDL is transporting cholesterol from the peripheries of the body back to the liver for breakdown and removal, it is considered good. This is misleading and unhelpful.

However, recommendations currently are that we should aim to reduce total cholesterol, as it has a role to play in the aetiology (set of causes) of cardiovascular disease, getting roped into normal repair mechanisms that take place when the endothelial wall (the inner lining of the blood vessels) is damaged.

Nutritional Therapy for High Cholesterol

Get carb smart

One area that is seldom discussed in relation to high cholesterol is the types of carbohydrates that we eat. Focus is so often on the fats in our diet. However, too many refined carbohydrates can make our cholesterol shoot up. White bread, white rice, white pasta, etc. release their sugars rapidly, as they have very little fibre and take little digestive effort to liberate these sugars.

This causes our blood sugar levels to rise significantly and rapidly. A certain amount of this can be shuttled to our cells to be used as energy. However, cells can only take in so much at one time and any excess is sent to the liver where it is converted into triacylglycerol – a type of fat that can eventually be stored as an energy source for a rainy day. When this is transported through our circulation, it causes a rise in LDL cholesterol.

Simply swapping over to multigrain or wholemeal versions of these staples can have a huge impact. They are far higher in fibre and take much longer to digest as a result. This liberates their sugars over a much longer period of time.

There is a second benefit: high-fibre whole grains have been clinically proven to lower cholesterol, and it is the fibre that is the key. These grains contain a lot of soluble fibre that forms a gel-like substance in the digestive tract. This binds to cholesterol within the gut (mostly from our liver via the bile), which then gets reabsorbed back into circulation in the intestine. By binding to soluble fibres like pectin and beta glucans, cholesterol cannot be reabsorbed and is, instead, carried away via the bowel.

Increase omega-3

Omega-3 fatty acids have been shown to improve the ratios between LDL and HDL cholesterol. Higher HDL and lower LDL has been linked with reduced risk of cardiovascular disease.

Top Foods

Low-GI carbohydrates	Omega-3
Oats	Salmon
Brown rice	Mackerel
Quinoa	Herring
Pearl barley	Fresh tuna
Bulgur wheat	

INSOMNIA

Insomnia is a common thing here in the UK, affecting around two-thirds of us at any one time. Around a third of us, according to NHS data, are experiencing this chronically or long term. In short, this condition is characterized by an inability to either fall asleep or stay asleep. We may lay awake for hours trying to get off to sleep. We may wake multiple times in the night and struggle to drift back off to sleep. It can also present as waking up too early in the morning and not feeling refreshed and rested from sleep.

For most of us, insomnia is just a temporary, annoying blip that troubles us for a day or two and then all is well. However, for those who experience chronic insomnia, the situation can be quite serious. Firstly, it can be a sign of other significant health issues such as depression and chronic stress. Prolonged sleep deprivation can drastically depress our immunity, causing white blood cell numbers to drop considerably, and it can increase cardiovascular disease risk and raise blood pressure. Secondly, it can also have endocrine effects (affecting glands that produce and secrete regulatory hormones), increasing the risk of type 2 diabetes and obesity.

Nutritional Therapy for Insomnia

General tips

Before we get to the specifics, there are a few tips that are relevant to everyone for getting a better night's sleep. The first is avoiding caffeine in the later part of the day. This should be fairly obvious, but caffeine, of course, is a stimulant, and while each of us has a varying tolerance to it, consumed after early afternoon it can keep us in a heightened state of alertness that can impact our ability to fall asleep. Therefore, I advise not consuming it after around 2pm, and instead opt for herbal teas.

The next thing is to avoid alcohol. Yes, I am the bearer of bad news, but alcohol, while it does indeed make us feel more relaxed and sleepy, once we begin to metabolize it, it causes a spike in the hormone cortisol, which wakes us up. This is the hormone that begins to rise in the morning to get us out of slumber. When this hormone spikes in the middle of the night, you will wake up and struggle to get back to sleep again.

Don't eat large meals right before bed. This isn't just one of those urban myths where apparently eating at night makes us gain weight. It's more a case of while we are trying to digest a big meal and many metabolic processes are running on high gear, we are not able to get into a fully rested state.

Increase magnesium intake

I know magnesium pops up a lot, but when it comes to a good night's sleep, it is an absolute hero nutrient. Firstly and most superficially, it can act as a muscle relaxant. If you are feeling tense and wound up and are holding a lot of tension in your muscles, this can get in the way of you being able to fully relax and get a decent sleep. Extra magnesium can help to relax the muscles and ease tension. More importantly, though, magnesium helps to elevate levels of GABA (gamma-aminobutyric acid) – the primary inhibitory neurotransmitter – and this means that it calms and slows things down.

There are many neurotransmitters with many roles to play. Some of them, such as glutamate, are excitatory, meaning they ramp up the nervous system and have a stimulatory effect, while others have the role of calming things down and relaxing the nervous system.

We are designed to have a peak of the excitatory neurotransmitters in the morning, plus the hormone cortisol to get us awake and ready to tackle the day. Then in the evening, we tend to get an increase in GABA to help us wind down, and when it gets dark, an elevation of melatonin production, which, when combined, get us off to sleep. However, with the stresses and strains of modern life we can easily get stuck in a state of elevated cortisol, overstimulation of the nervous system and low levels of GABA. This leads to a racing mind, agitation, irritability and an inability to relax.

In this situation, I recommend both food sources of magnesium and a supplement. Make sure that you load up on green leafy vegetables in your evening meal, as these are the richest food sources of magnesium. Think kale, cavolo nero, spring greens or broccoli. Supplement-wise, taking around 400mg 30 minutes before you go to bed is adequate.

Eat tryptophan-rich foods

Tryptophan is a naturally occurring amino acid that will cross the blood-brain barrier and be converted into the neuro-transmitter serotonin, known as the feel-good neurotransmitter. At night, when the brain perceives darkness, serotonin is then converted into a hormone called melatonin, and this chemical sets sleep patterns and can help us to get a deeper, longer sleep.

Dietary sources of tryptophan, when consumed with a good-quality carbohydrate, can be very helpful in getting us off to sleep and keeping us there. This combination is important, as we need a gentle insulin spike to catapult the tryptophan across the blood-brain barrier. So think along the lines of a small tuna open sandwich, a mini turkey wrap or a banana and some peanut butter combined. Just ensure the serving is small and that the carbohydrate is a low-glycaemic multigrain source.

BEST FOOD SOURCES OF TRYPTOPHAN
- Turkey
- Tuna
- Salmon
- Spinach
- Nuts

Increase the Bs, but at the right time

The final group of nutrients that are particularly important are the B vitamins, but it is important that we take them at the right time. The B vitamins are absolutely vital for the manufacture of all neurotransmitters, serotonin included, and don't forget that serotonin is the precursor to melatonin, which sets the clock, so we need to ensure abundant serotonin levels to begin with. B vitamins also regulate many aspects of neurological function and can help us to cope with stress more effectively, as well as reducing the levels of the hormone cortisol, which can play havoc with our sleep cycles.

A daily supplement is likely to be your best bet here, such as a B50 or B100 complex. However, you must take them in the earlier part of the day with either breakfast or lunch. This is simply because they are vital for turning food into energy. They facilitate the cellular conversion of glucose into adenosine triphosphate (ATP), the fuel for our cells, and while they are not a stimulant, they *can* make you feel very energized, so many people struggle to get to sleep when they take B vitamins in the evening.

IRRITABLE BOWEL SYNDROME (IBS)

Irritable bowel syndrome (IBS) is an issue that plagues millions globally, and is something that has no clearly defined cause. It is essentially a collection of different symptoms that can manifest in a wide variety of ways. Symptoms include constipation, diarrhoea, bloating (trapped wind), intestinal cramps and gas. There are many potential triggers for some individuals, and these are often unique to the person.

However, there is one intervention that has become incredibly successful globally, and that is the FODMAP diet. FODMAP stands for 'fermentable oligosaccharides, disaccharides, monosaccharides and polyols'. These are basically very large, complex sugars that are not digested in the small intestine the way the more simple sugars are. They are intact throughout the small intestine and reach the large intestine whole, causing much more work for the large intestine. This is the key to their ability to cause symptoms in susceptible individuals.

In some individuals, when FODMAPs are in the small intestine they can rapidly draw water into the small intestine, which causes the walls to stretch. Stretch receptors are then stimulated, which causes rapid, forceful contractions, and the result is large-volume watery diarrhoea that comes on with intense urgency. In others, the FODMAPs don't create any kind of issue in the small intestine; instead, they cause havoc in the large intestine. Any sugars that don't get broken down in the small intestine will be set upon by the gut flora, the bacterial colony that live in the gut, which begin to break them down by means of fermentation. Now for most of us, this fermentation process will help support the bacterial colony by helping it to flourish. It will also cause the release of several by-products that can support gut health in many ways. However, in individuals sensitive to FODMAPs, this fermentation process produces masses of gas, which leads to severe bloating, cramps and gas.

Nutritional Therapy for IBS

Reduce high-FODMAP foods

There is a chart for you here to make it a little easier choosing foods, but some examples of high-FODMAP foods are apples, mangoes, pears, most soft or unpasteurized dairy products, chickpeas (garbanzo beans), lentils, beans, artichokes, asparagus, cauliflower, onions, garlic and leeks. This is just a selection and the chart will give you the bigger picture.

Base your diet around low-FODMAP foods

Again, the chart will give you a more complete list, but low FODMAP foods include bananas, blueberries, grapes, carrots, corn, celery and hard cheeses.

Grains & Pulses	Nuts & Seeds	Other
Oats	Almonds	Butter
Polenta	Hazelnuts	Eggs
Quinoa	Peanuts	Hard cheeses
Rice (white)	Pumpkin seeds	Maple syrup (small amount)
	Sesame seeds	Non-dairy milks
	Sunflower seeds	
	Walnuts	

Vegetables	Fruit
Artichokes	Bananas
Aubergines (eggplants)	Blueberries
Broccoli	Cranberries
Butternut squash	Grapefruit
Cabbage	Grapes
Carrots	Kiwi fruit
Celery	Lemons & limes
Corn (small amount)	Melon
Courgettes (zucchini)	Oranges
Green beans	Passionfruit
Kale	Pineapple
Olives	Raspberries
Parsnips	Rhubarb
Peppers (bell peppers)	Strawberries
Potatoes	
Pumpkin	
Spinach	
Sweet potatoes	
Tomatoes	

LOW LIBIDO AND IMPAIRED SEXUAL FUNCTION

This is an issue that so few people talk about, but it is something that is on the rise (perhaps a bad choice of words there!). There are three main drivers for this – emotional issues, hormonal issues and blood flow.

Emotional issues, such as anxiety and depression, have been very closely linked with lack of libido and reduced sexual function. This seems especially true in men where emotions can directly influence the activity of the sexual organs. Anxiety and stress are some of the most common causes of reduced sexual function in men, less so in women.

Hormonal issues are some of the trickiest to tackle in this context. This is because hormonal changes and fluctuations are really just related to age, and there is only so much we can do about that. However, sometimes diet can influence this. We know, for example, that insulin resistance can cause PCOS (polycystic ovary syndrome) and increase androgen production in women, and being overweight can reduce testosterone and increase oestrogen in men, so lifestyle can impact this.

The aspect that is easiest to manipulate with dietary intervention is blood flow to the sexual organs. For both men and women, blood flow to the sexual organs is absolutely vital for arousal and for proper penetrative sex to occur. Impaired blood flow reduces clitoral sensitivity and vaginal lubrication, and, of course, will impair a proper erection. The good news is, however, that food can certainly influence this quite considerably.

Nutritional Therapy for Low Libido and Impaired Sexual Function

Reduce anxiety with magnesium and B vitamins

Obviously, so many factors influence anxiety and I'm not going to pretend that a bit of magnesium is the answer to everything, but certainly a few important nutrients can minimize the severity of anxiety. The first is magnesium because it helps to increase the production of a neurotransmitter called GABA (gamma-aminobutyric acid), the primary inhibitory neurotransmitter, which is the brain chemical that helps to calm everything down. When the mind is racing at a million miles an hour, GABA helps to bring everything back to a calm state.

The B vitamins are vital for the manufacture of neuro-transmitters, and in their own right have quite a relaxing effect upon the nervous system by regulating many key functions.

BEST FOOD SOURCES OF MAGNESIUM

- Cavolo nero
- Kale
- Spring greens
- Broccoli
- Nuts and seeds
- Pulses (legumes)

BEST FOOD SOURCES OF B VITAMINS

- Whole grains
- Nuts
- Seeds
- Green vegetables
- Pulses (legumes)
- Yeast extract
- Beef
- Chicken

Keep hormones in check

Okay, so as I have alluded to, there are many reasons why hormones can be out of whack. Quite simply, the most common hormonal link with low libido and impaired sexual function is ageing. As we age, many of the hormones that would have us raring to go in the bedroom just begin to deplete. In men, testosterone begins to decline just past the age of 30. In women, once the menopause is in full swing, oestrogen levels begin to plummet. A drop in both of these hormones can exacerbate anxiety and depression, cause low energy levels, negatively affect sexual organ function and put you as far away from 'in the mood' as you can imagine. Now, these age-related hormonal declines can be slowed down by a lifetime of eating healthily, doing plenty of exercise, getting good sleep and good stress management, but even if you live like Yoda, it will get you eventually.

There are, however, a few incidences where our diet and lifestyle can create internal biochemical and metabolic changes that mimic some of these age-related hormonal changes. The first, for men in particular, is being overweight. This is because when we are carrying additional body fat, we have high levels of an enzyme called aromatase, which can convert testosterone into oestrogen. This means that our testosterone levels plummet faster, and at the same time oestrogen levels rise. The falling testosterone will affect libido and erectile function, and the raised oestrogen can increase our risk of some cancers. So doing whatever you can to lose some weight is a big priority.

In women, there is a very, very strong link between continually high levels of insulin and impaired ovarian function, to the extent that PCOS (polycystic ovary syndrome) can develop. When ovaries are cystic, eggs are not released, corpus luteum formation doesn't occur and natural oestrogen production begins to decline. As you have seen elsewhere in this book, keeping insulin down is achieved by managing blood sugar effectively. To do this, first avoid the simple sugars such as those found in confectionery, swap your carb staples such as rice, bread, etc., to the brown wholegrain versions and cut down on your portion sizes of these, then when you do eat them, always combine them with a really good protein source and a lot of non-starchy vegetables (see page 105).

Enhance blood flow with flavonoids

Enhancing blood flow is the aspect of reduced sexual function that we can really influence from a dietary perspective, with one group of phytochemicals having a notable impact, namely the flavonoids. Found in foods such as green tea, chocolate, berries and red wine, flavonoids are colour pigments, and it has been discovered that they can be taken up by the endothelial cells, which make up the skin that lines the inside of our blood vessels. When flavonoids are taken up by this skin, they cause metabolic distress within the cells that induces them to start expressing high levels of a gas called nitric oxide. The nitric oxide then leaves the endothelial cells and moves out into the smooth muscle that makes up the blood vessel walls, causing the fibres to relax. As the fibres relax, the vessel dilates and gets bigger, and as it gets bigger, blood flow improves.

MENOPAUSE

The menopause is a very distressing time of transition for many, whereas for others it can be a relatively smooth ride. It can manifest in so many ways with such a varying intensity. It is due to a gradual reduction in ovarian function. As the ovaries begin to lose normal function, there is a corresponding variation in normal hormone profiles. When this happens, the brain tries to compensate by releasing other hormones. This mixed-up hormonal profile causes havoc in the body and can result in a whole host of symptoms, from hot flushes and weight gain, even through to depression and hair loss.

Nutritional Therapy for Menopause

Diet CAN play a role in managing the menopause, but this is certainly one time when we need to look at diet as a PART of the picture here.

Focus on phytoestrogens

Phytoestrogens are a group of chemicals that resemble an almost identical chemical structure to oestrogen that the body produces. So similar, in fact, that they can actually bind to oestrogen receptors on cells, but they don't actually instigate the response that oestrogen does (see page 66).

In cases like the menopause, these substances can be incredibly useful. Many of the symptoms that are experienced during the menopause arise when hormone levels, particularly oestrogen, drop and the receptors start to freak out. For the same reason that people get cravings when they are addicted to nicotine, the receptors – when they don't get their fix – create a whole sequence of chaotic signals that cause many of the symptoms associated with the menopause. Phytoestrogens, by binding to the receptors, can appease their cravings for hormonal interaction.

Focus on skeletal support

Skeletal density does naturally begin to decline from around the age of 35, but as soon as the menopause kicks in, this process accelerates and bone density declines more rapidly, so supporting skeletal health is of vital importance. This will mean a focus on a few individual nutrients.

We hear so much about increasing intake of calcium, but without a host of other nutrients, calcium can't be utilized. I like to use the analogy of bricks on a building site. Sure they are the structural material, but without a team of builders nothing will happen to it. Likewise, without vitamin D and magnesium, calcium intake is meaningless. We need these additional nutrients to get it into the skeleton.

Increase omega-3 fatty acid intake

One area that also becomes a point of concern for menopausal women is an increased risk of cardiovascular disease. Omega-3 fatty acids help to improve HDL to LDL cholesterol ratios (see page 83), reduce inflammation within blood vessels and also reduce excessive clotting, so are a great long-term prophylactic (defence) against cardiovascular disease.

Top Foods

Phytoestrogen-rich foods	Calcium-rich foods
Miso	Green leafy vegetables
Tempeh	Cashew nuts
Chickpeas (garbanzo beans)	Dairy products
Flaxseeds (linseeds)	Sunflower seeds
	Fortified dairy alternatives, e.g. soya

Magnesium-rich foods

Dark green vegetables –
the greener the better

Figs

Avocado

Nuts and seeds

Vitamin D-rich foods

Full-fat dairy products

Oily fish

Vitamin D-enriched
mushrooms (special variety
in supermarkets)

MIGRAINE

Migraines can vary from the bad through to the utterly debilitating. Symptoms can range from intense headaches to sickness, disturbed vision, flashes of light and even physical sickness. Migraines are beyond just headaches: they are, in fact, a neurological disorder that has been linked to serotonin levels. Low serotonin levels can produce blood vessel disturbances in the brain: when they contract they can cause visual disturbances, then when they relax they cause the headaches. This continual excessive contraction and dilation is what results in the problem. While the exact causes of this are unknown, there have been certain triggers identified in some individuals. These could be stress, alcohol and even particular foods.

Nutritional Therapy for Migraine

Cut back on common triggers
The triggers could potentially be anything in anyone, but the commonly identified ones are caffeine, red wine and chocolate. Other acknowledged triggers are shellfish, nuts and seeds, spices and sugar. There are also some reports that the flavour enhancer MSG (monosodium glutamate), commonly found in Chinese food, may be a trigger. It really can be trial and error in discovering your personal trigger, and there is no sprecific prescriptive plan to follow.

Try magnesium oil
There is some good evidence that magnesium oil applied to the upper part of the neck at the base of the skull during an attack can noticeably reduce the length and severity of the attack.

MUSCLE CRAMPS

I hate these. Out of nowhere that tightening and burning pain cuts through you! It is a sudden, involuntary, forceful contraction of a muscle that can range from slight discomfort to absolute agony. Muscle cramps can be caused by many things, including overexertion, prolonged tension, dehydration and low levels of key nutrients. While most cramps are harmless, there are occasions where they can be the sign of something more serious, like reduced blood flow, so if you experience ongoing cramp in the same area, then make sure you see your doctor.

Nutritional Therapy for Muscle Cramps

Magnesium two ways

Magnesium really is the king of cramp treatments, for the simple reason that it is the nutrient directly involved in muscular relaxation. Calcium and magnesium work in tandem to control muscular contraction and relaxation. Calcium flows into muscle cells and causes muscle fibres to contract, and conversely, when magnesium flows in, muscle fibres relax.

Increasing magnesium in the diet can be a great tool for the prevention of cramps. I would advise getting it in at every meal. It is richest in green leafy vegetables, so if it is green, it is magnesium rich! This is all thanks to chlorophyll, and magnesium forms a key part of the chlorophyll structure.

BEST FOOD SOURCES OF MAGNESIUM
- Cavolo nero
- Kale
- Spring greens
- Broccoli
- Nuts and seeds
- Pulses (legumes)

Getting more magnesium in the diet is a good preventer, but what about treatment? Well, popping a supplement can mean that the nutrient won't get into circulation and be delivered where needed for a good couple of hours. In the throes of a muscle cramp attack, topical magnesium therapy hits the spot, so this means applying magnesium oil directly to the affected area so that it will rapidly move transdermally (through the skin) to the locked-up muscle and help it to gently relax.

NAUSEA

Nausea is essentially a symptom. It isn't a condition or an issue in its own right, but a symptom that has arisen for myriad different potential reasons. Travel sickness, morning sickness, hangovers and overeating are all relatively minor reasons for nausea to rear its head. However, there are also serious issues, such as liver disease, that can feature nausea as part of their symptomology, so of course, if it is going on for a long time, go and see your doctor.

Nutritional Therapy for Nausea

Eat bitter foods

One of the oldest and most traditional ways of treating nausea is with bitters. Herbs like gentian, for example, were the go-tos, and there is scientific validity here (which isn't always the case with traditional remedies). When our tongue detects a bitter flavour, there is a stimulation of the vagus and hypoglossal nerves, and this, in turn, increases secretion of gastric juices and the release of bile, both of which can ease transient nausea.

Sip on ginger tea

Another of the traditional remedies for nausea is to take ginger, either served as a tea, eaten as crystallized (candied) ginger or even juiced fresh ginger; a good dose of the spicy stuff can help to ease nausea. The volatile oils that give ginger its spicy flavour help to relax the gastric walls. It also appears that, in a similar way to bitters, ginger helps to regulate gastric secretions.

OSTEOPOROSIS

Osteoporosis is, in MOST cases, a disease of advancing years, although there are some rare exceptions. It is, in essence, a loss of bone density that gets so severe that it noticeably increases the risk of fractures.

The decline in bone density is a perfectly normal thing that begins at around 35 years of age. However, some lifestyle choices can influence how rapidly and the extent to which this happens. Lack of exercise, being over- or underweight and restrictive diets can accelerate the process. When we get to a certain stage in life, the bone density loss can speed up further. Women are at greater risk at the time of the menopause. Oestrogen helps to maintain bone density, so as this drops, it will accelerate the natural process of bone loss.

Nutritional Therapy for Osteoporosis

Support bone-protecting calcium absorption with vitamin D
Vitamin D has been spoken about so much in recent years and is the hot nutrient of the moment. The primary function of vitamin D is to maintain serum concentrations of calcium. When we consume calcium-rich foods and our blood levels of calcium rise, vitamin D takes it out of circulation and delivers it to the skeleton. For decades we have had it drummed into us that we need to consume calcium for healthy bones. Well, that is only part of the picture. I like to use the analogy of bricks on the building site. Sure they are the structural material, but without builders nothing will happen. Well, vitamin D is one of the most important builders you can get to actually do something with the calcium and get it to where it needs to go.

Magnesium

Magnesium is one of the most commonly deficient nutrients in this country, and is one of the most important because it is involved in over 1,000 chemical reactions in the body. It is another of the vital builders on the skeletal building site. It is required for the formation of calcitriol, which is the active form of vitamin D. Adequate magnesium intake helps to reduce the release of the parathyroid hormone (PTH), which increases calcium loss from the skeleton.

Top Foods

Vitamin D	Magnesium
Full-fat dairy products	Green leafy vegetables
Oily fish	Pulses (legumes)
Vitamin D-enriched mushrooms (special variety in supermarkets)	Oily fish
	Nuts and seeds
	Dark chocolate

POLYCYSTIC OVARY SYNDROME (PCOS)

PCOS is characterized by the formation of a series of cysts upon the ovary, where eggs have not formed properly during the cycle. Normally, when an egg forms, it gradually moves towards the membranous lining of the ovary and pops through it to head into the fallopian tube. When this happens, a small sac is left behind that secretes hormones that regulate the menstrual cycle. When PCOS occurs, the egg is unable to break free from the ovary and forms a cyst. This cyst creates higher than normal androgen hormones (the precursors to oestrogen), which can cause symptoms such as acne and hirsutism (facial hair).

Nutritional Therapy for PCOS

Maintain stable blood sugar levels

There is a strong link between a high-glycaemic diet, i.e. one that raises blood sugar too high for too long, and the development of PCOS. Choose a lower-carbohydrate diet, building it around good-quality proteins, fats and non-starchy vegetables such as alfalfa, celery, asparagus, spinach and lettuce. Any carbohydrates you do eat, opt for wholegrain varieties and take the portion sizes that you eat down to less than half of what you would normally consume, but the focus needs to be on the proteins, fats and non-starchy veg.

Increase omega-3 fatty acids

Increasing omega-3 fatty acids will help to tone down inflammation, which is a common feature of PCOS.

Eat walnuts and almonds

Regular consumption of these nuts can help lower androgen hormones (see above).

Increase zinc-rich foods

Zinc is also vital in the metabolism and breakdown of androgen hormones. These are the hormones, like testosterone, that we commonly associate with men. They can affect follicular formation within the ovaries, stimulate the sebaceous glands and trigger acne.

Top Foods

Omega-3
Salmon
Mackerel
Herring
Anchovies
Pollock

Zinc-rich foods
Prawns (shrimp)
Walnuts
Pumpkin seeds
Oily fish

PSORIASIS

Psoriasis is a skin disorder that is becoming increasingly common. It is one that centres around the turnover of new skin cells. These are formed at the very bottom layer of our skin, and gradually make their way outwards as the cells above them die and fall off.

In psoriasis, this process becomes accelerated and occurs at an unregulated rate. It may well be that this is triggered by some kind of autoimmune event whereby the immune system begins to attack some of the body's own tissues. In this case, it occurs in the lower layers of the skin, affecting skin cell turnover as a result. It is believed that certain cell lines within the immune system cause localized inflammatory damage that produces the initial redness and irritation that sufferers experience during the early stages of a flare-up. This results in an accelerated die-off of skin cells.

As the inflammation eases, the lesion becomes dry and scaly with a distinctive silvery appearance to the flaking skin.

Nutritional Therapy for Psoriasis

Increase omega-3

As you have probably noted by now, omega-3 fatty acids provide the body with the building blocks that it needs to manufacture its own in-built anti-inflammatory compounds. The early stages of psoriasis involve acute inflammatory episodes. If inflammation can be eased even to a small degree, this can make a significant difference to the severity of the flare-up. It doesn't take away the condition, but it makes flare-ups less angry.

Eat more orange foods

Foods such as sweet potatoes, carrots and mangoes are all rich in fat-soluble antioxidants such as beta carotene, responsible for their orange-coloured pigment. This class of antioxidant can accumulate in the skin and offer localized anti-inflammatory activity. The redness and irritation at the beginning of a psoriasis flare-up is active inflammation. Anything you can do to reduce this will lessen the severity of the lesion, and an ample intake of carotenoids can help with this.

Top Foods

Omega-3
Salmon
Mackerel
Herring
Fresh tuna

Carotenoid-rich foods
Sweet potatoes
Mangoes
Carrots

RESTLESS LEGS SYNDROME

Restless legs syndrome (RLS), also known as Willis-Ekbom disease, is a troublesome condition that causes discomfort and strange sensations in the legs together with an intense urge to move them, especially at night. Exact causes aren't fully understood, but there are nutritional links. Primary RLS is thought in some way to be related to dopamine. Secondary RLS, however, is more often a complication of other issues, including nutritional deficiencies.

Nutritional Therapy for Restless Legs Syndrome

Increase iron intake

One of the main theories around restless legs is that there is either a lack of iron or that the brain is not using iron correctly. This could well be from a simple lack of iron intake, or be related to more serious underlying issues like kidney disease, but in most cases, it's a simple dietary deficiency. The link here is that iron is responsible for oxygen delivery to tissues, as it is a key part of red blood cells bound to haemoglobin. Poor circulation and/or poor delivery of oxygen to tissues are key features of restless legs syndrome. Iron also has a link with dopamine synthesis. Therefore, the first step is to up your iron intake, and iron-rich foods go way beyond just red meat, so focus on spinach, kale, dried apricots and beans and pulses (legumes).

Increase magnesium intake

Extra magnesium can help to relax the muscles and ease tension, and can reduce the urge to keep moving. More importantly, though, magnesium helps to elevate levels of GABA – the primary inhibitory neurotransmitter – and this means that it calms and slows things down.

There are many neurotransmitters with many roles to play – see Nutritional Therapy for Insomnia starting on page 85. Increasing magnesium can help to increase this calming effect by raising GABA, and it has the double whammy of also being a muscle relaxant.

I recommend taking a supplement of 400mg magnesium daily about an hour before you go to bed.

RICKETS AND OSTEOMALACIA

Rickets is something that used to be very common 50–60 years ago but had been as good as wiped out. Now, however, it is starting to rear its ugly head again. Rickets occurs when there has been insufficient mineralization around the collagen framework on which bone is built. In gestation and infancy, bones start off as a firm gel-like structure that take on minerals to turn them hard. Our body relies on vitamin D to take calcium out of the bloodstream, get it to the skeleton and stimulate bone-building cells called osteoblasts to lay it down and harden it. A vitamin D deficiency, therefore, leads to bones that are not strong enough to bear the weight of the growing child and the bones bow.

Osteomalacia is the same condition in adults. Both of these conditions are related to low vitamin D levels. This, in turn, reduces the amount of calcium that gets into the skeleton, making bones begin to soften. So why has this started to appear again? Well, the primary source of vitamin D for humans is the conversion of cholesterol into vitamin D precursors within the skin upon exposure to ultra violet radiation (UV rays), i.e. sunshine. In the UK and other northerly parts of the world, we have relatively little of that, and when we do, we slather on vast amounts of super-high-SPF sunscreens. This means that we are unable to synthesize vitamin D when the sun does come out.

Nutritional Therapy for Rickets and Osteomalacia

Increase vitamin D intake

There really is only one real way to tackle rickets and osteomalacia head on, and that is to drastically increase vitamin D intake. Vitamin D is the nutrient that takes calcium from our circulation and lays it down in the skeleton.

Top Foods

Full-fat dairy products

Oily fish

Vitamin D-enriched mushrooms
(special variety in supermarkets)

URINARY TRACT INFECTIONS (UTI)

Urinary tract infections are normal and common, and, apart from being uncomfortable, are quite harmless. They occur when bacteria, notably *E. coli*, begin to embed themselves in the urethra and the bladder. The result is an immune response that leads to inflammation, which we experience as pain when passing water, ongoing irritation and the feeling of urinary urgency. Even though there is more frequent urination, there may be less volume; the irritation is what causes the need to go.

Nutritional Therapy for UTIs

Increase zinc intake

One of the key ways that nutrition can assist you in the case of a urinary tract infection is by supporting immunity to help clear the infection faster. One nutrient that really does have a good track record for doing this is zinc. This is because zinc is used by the white blood cells of the immune system to manufacture genes that actually control how effectively and aggressively they will respond to pathogens and infection. I recommend taking around 15mg of zinc daily for women, and around 30mg daily for men, in supplement form.

Increase omega-3 intake

This recommendation is really just to help ease the symptoms a little. Additional omega-3 in the diet, when coming from EPA and DHA found in oily fish or supplements, can actually increase the expression of substances called series 1 and series 3 prostaglandins that have a notable anti-inflammatory effect in the body. Much of the symptom pattern we experience during a UTI is coming from inflammation, so anything we can do to ease this will make us feel much more comfortable. Top up on oily fish like salmon, mackerel and herring to dose up on EPA and DHA.

Double down on fluid intake (mechanical movement)

Okay, so this recommendation may sound somewhat counter-intuitive. Urination is uncomfortable in the full throws of a UTI, so why would you want to pee more? Well, the mechanical movement can help to dislodge bacteria that has embedded within the urethra, and the motion of urine running through can help to mechanically remove bacteria. Aim to drink water to the point where you urinate four to six times per hour. While this isn't ideal for ongoing daily consumption, for this purpose it can be of great benefit.

Cranberry juice

Probably the most well known of all of the home remedies for treating UTIs is, of course, cranberry juice. While the extent of its ability to benefit may be somewhat overplayed, it does deliver some help and this is due to the presence of specific flavonoids within the fruit that can actually prevent bacteria from adhering to the walls of the urethra. It is best consumed at the very early signs of a UTI, and can even be considered as a food or supplement to consume regularly for those that get frequent UTIs. Supplements will certainly provide the most powerful effect, as the flavonoids will be concentrated in an extract.

Probiotics

A final option, specifically for women, is a daily probiotic to maintain the health and diversity of the vaginal flora that can increase defences against localized infection. There are two specific strains that have been studied in relation to urinary tract infections and have been shown to reach the vaginal flora and support it. These strains are *Lactobacillus rhamnosus* GR-1 and *Lactobacillus reuteri* RC-14. These need to be seen as a preventative rather than an intervention.

A–Z of Medicinal Foods

When you are referring to individual ingredients in this section of the book and you read 'good for', this doesn't mean that eating a couple of these ingredients will suddenly heal every condition imaginable. This is to highlight nutrients or phytochemical components that are relevant in certain conditions, to give you an idea of how you can make dietary changes to support your health. It has nothing to do with being an alternative to anything, but everything to do with empowerment.

ADZUKI BEANS

I love adzuki beans. These red beans are super versatile.

GOOD FOR
- Antioxidant intake
- Stabilizing blood sugar

Antioxidant intake

All beans are nutritional powerhouses, but adzuki beans pack a few extra punches with their antioxidant content. This is all thanks to polyphenols, the substances responsible for the adzuki beans' red skin colouring. Polyphenols are found in antioxidant-rich foods like green tea, red wine, berries, etc.

Stabilizing blood sugar

Adzuki beans, like all pulses (legumes), are very high in fibre, which is of vital importance in stabilizing blood sugar. This is because the high fibre content means that the food is digested far more slowly, releasing its sugars over a more gradual time period. This drip-feeds our blood sugar rather than drastically flooding it, keeping blood sugar levels far more stable.

OTHER BENEFITS
Rich in B vitamins

BEST WAY TO EAT
In stews, dips, spreads, mixed with other pulses (legumes)

ALMONDS

Roasted almonds. Almond butter. Whatever form they are in,
I absolutely adore almonds, and they make a very nutritious
snack indeed.

> **GOOD FOR**
> ➤ Healthy skin
> ➤ Cardiovascular health

Healthy skin

Almonds can pack a double whammy of benefits for the skin.
Firstly, they are rich in vitamin E, which is a fat-soluble
antioxidant, meaning that it has an affinity for fatty substances
and tissues. As such, it can help to protect skin cell membranes
from oxidative damage, and this helps to slow down certain
cellular ageing processes. It also keeps the cell membranes far
healthier and more flexible, which gives the skin softness and
suppleness. Vitamin E will also deliver some degree of localized
anti-inflammatory activity.

Almonds have a second way of benefiting our skin. They
are rich in the mineral zinc, and this is used by our sebaceous
glands to regulate oil secretions. If the skin is too oily or too dry,
adequate zinc in the diet can even things out. Zinc is also vital
for acne, as it supports immune function. Zinc is used by the
white blood cells of the immune system to manufacture genes
that regulate the way in which they respond to pathogens and
infection, and this helps to clear infection faster.

Cardiovascular health

Vitamin E is also an important nutrient for a healthy
cardiovascular system. As a fat-soluble antioxidant, it can
help to prevent oxidation of cholesterol and blood lipids (fats).

Oxidation of these substances plays a key role in the instigation of cardiovascular disease (see page 229).

BEST WAY TO EAT

Ground on cereals, as an almond butter or just eaten whole, preferably raw

APPLES

We all know that old phrase of an apple a day keeping the doctor away. Bit of a cliché that's true, but there are some properties in this simple daily staple that are certainly impressive for such a cheap food item.

GOOD FOR
- Heart health
- Digestion and gut flora support
- Antioxidant intake

Heart health

Apples are very rich in a type of soluble fibre called pectin (jam makers may know of this stuff already). This fibre takes on many times its own weight in water, causing it to swell up and form a gel-like substance in the gut. When this gel-like substance forms, it binds to cholesterol in the gut, trapping it, and then carries it away via the bowel. This cholesterol is not from food; it is released by the liver during digestion and gets reabsorbed later on. This binding by pectin prevents it from being absorbed, so blood levels begin to go down. Regular consumption of pectin-rich foods can significantly reduce cholesterol.

Antioxidant intake

I think it's pretty hard to find a fruit or vegetable that isn't antioxidant rich. Apples aren't exactly the most powerful when we compare it to foods like blueberries for example, but what they do have is a diverse range of antioxidant compounds. For example, the red-skinned varieties contain anthocyanins – part of the chemistry that produces the colour pigment. These have extensive benefits for cardiovascular health (see blueberries, page 132, for more information). They contain catechins like

those found in green tea (see page 121); quercetin, which has
an anti-inflammatory activity, and chlorogenic acid, known to
support liver health. Don't worry about every single compound
– the take-home from this really is that you don't have to spend
a fortune on weird and wonderful ingredients to eat healthily –
simple everyday staples are just as nutritious.

OTHER BENEFITS

Apples are also rich in vitamin C, biotin (see page 216)
and magnesium

BEST WAY TO EAT

Eaten fresh, juiced, lightly baked

APRICOTS

I am a great fan of apricots. They just don't seem to show up on the shelves as much as they used to. When I do see them, I snap them up.

> **GOOD FOR**
> - Skin health
> - Anti-inflammatory boost
> - Heart health

Skin health

Probably the greatest nutritional nugget found in apricots is beta carotene. This is what gives them their distinctive orange colour. Beta carotene is a fat-soluble antioxidant, meaning that it will naturally migrate into fatty tissues. Second to the brain, the most abundant fatty tissue in the body is the subcutaneous layer of the skin. Fat-soluble antioxidants such as beta carotene can begin to accumulate in the subcutaneous layer and offer localized antioxidant protection, helping to protect structures such as collagen and elastin from damage. This, over time, can protect against accelerated ageing of the skin.

Anti-inflammatory boost

Apricots are a rich source of antioxidant compounds called catechins that are found in other food stuffs such as green tea. Catechins have been shown to reduce the activity of an enzyme called cyclo-oxygenase that is responsible for creating substances in the body that switch on the inflammatory response. By interfering with this enzyme, inflammatory load is lessened.

Heart health

As these little gems are rich in beta carotene (see Skin Health on the previous page), they have a specific ability to reduce the incidence of lipid (blood fat) oxidation. This means they can prevent the oxidation of cholesterol and triglycerides (where they react with oxygen and can potentially become toxic) – events that cause damage to the endothelium that lines the inside of blood vessels. This damage then sets forth a cascade of responses that can eventually lead to arterial plaque associated with heart disease. Keeping this damage at bay in the first place is a key preventative measure.

OTHER BENEFITS

Rich in quercetin and dietary fibre

BEST WAY TO EAT

Eaten fresh or use to add thickness and silkiness to smoothies

ARTICHOKES

This giant, edible flower is a food shrouded in mystery –
certainly in the UK. Artichokes are a commonly used vegetable
across the Mediterranean and have crossed from the culinary
realm into the world of botanical medicine. I love them in pasta
dishes or cooked with capers and shallots with some white fish.

GOOD FOR
- Liver health
- Digestive health

Liver health

In botanical medicine, artichokes have long gained a reputation
as being a remedy for liver health. Recent research has given
some potential scientific validity to this. One particular
substance identified in artichokes, caffeoylquinic acid, can
have a noticeable anti-inflammatory effect on the liver. It is
also known to increase the flow of bile, which can help in the
removal of substances that have been converted into harmless,
fat-soluble substances ready for excretion from the body.

Digestive health

The way in which artichokes can benefit digestive health, aside
from being high in dietary fibre, is the effect they have upon
bile flow, as mentioned above. Bile serves two main roles: as the
transport system for broken-down waste products and for the
digestion of fats. If you have ever poured oil on water, you will
know that the oil sits on the surface in giant globules. Well, the
same thing occurs in the digestive system when we consume
fats. These giant globules cannot be absorbed in such a state,
so they have to be emulsified, i.e. broken down into tiny droplets
that can then be absorbed via specialist absorption sites within

the digestive tract. Bile is the substance the body uses to perform this task, emulsifying fats into small droplets ready for absorption. Bile is also what could be considered the body's own in-built laxative, helping the movement of gut contents on their way.

OTHER BENEFITS

Artichokes are high in dietary fibre, which gives general support to gut and cardiovascular health

BEST WAY TO EAT

Artichoke hearts in salads and pasta dishes, or sautéed in garlic as a side dish; whole artichokes stuffed with brown rice or quinoa

ASPARAGUS

Asparagus is one of those vegetables that is considered a bit 'posh'. Not quite sure where that reputation comes from, as during the summer months it is a very abundant crop in the UK. I absolutely love it with a couple of poached eggs and some Hollandaise sauce. Heaven.

GOOD FOR
➥ Urinary health

Urinary health
Asparagus can help to increase urinary flow by acting as a gentle irritant to the filtration system of the kidney – the nephron. This gentle irritation causes a diuretic-like action, which can be useful in issues such as urinary tract infections, where increased urination can help to dislodge infectious bacteria. It can also be helpful in water retention. There is a tell-tale sign when asparagine is active and doing its thing – the distinct smell of asparagus urine. Unpleasant, yes, but a sign that it is active.

OTHER BENEFITS
There is some evidence to suggest that a substance in asparagus called racemofuran can have a mild anti-inflammatory effect

BEST WAY TO EAT
Lightly cooked or steamed, or eaten raw, cut into thin ribbons, in a salad

AUBERGINES (EGGPLANTS)

The humble aubergine is one of my favourites of the Mediterranean staple vegetables. It is so versatile and is a real flavour sponge.

GOOD FOR
- Digestive health
- Healthy nervous system

Digestive health

Aubergines are very high in dietary fibre. This benefits digestive health in two ways. Firstly, dietary fibre takes on many times its own weight in water within the digestive tract. This causes it to swell greatly, stretching the gut wall, in turn activating so-called 'stretch receptors' that then stimulate contraction of the gut wall, moving everything along. Dietary fibre also supports the growth and flourishing of the gut flora colony that lives inside the gut and supports many aspects of health.

Healthy nervous system

Some newer research has suggested that aubergines may help support the health of the nervous system. This is due to the substance that gives it its deep black/purple colour – nasunin. It is believed that nasunin can help to protect the fatty lining of nerve cells from damage.

BEST WAY TO EAT
I especially like them in a ratatouille or stuffed and baked; they also make a good alternative to pasta sheets in lasagne

AVOCADOS

People often think these little powerhouses are unhealthy because of their high oil content. But do yourself a favour and add them to your diet wherever possible. You will be glad that you did!

GOOD FOR
- High cholesterol
- Skin health
- Heart and circulation

High cholesterol

Avocados are very high in a fatty acid called oleic acid, also found in olive oil, which many trials have shown causes a reduction in 'bad' (LDL) cholesterol, and a subtle increase in 'good' (HDL) cholesterol.

Skin health

Avocados are also very high in the fat-soluble antioxidant vitamin E. This helps protect skin cell membranes from chemical damage, and can be an important part of a natural skincare regime.

Heart and circulation

The high vitamin E content of avocado makes it a wonderful food for heart health. Vitamin E is a natural anticoagulant, meaning it reduces blood-clotting activity and may offer protective benefit against heart attack and stroke.

BEST WAY TO EAT
Mashed on toast, chopped in salads, made into guacamole

BANANAS

Probably the most widely eaten fruit on the planet, and one that you can get even the most hardcore plant dodger to eat most of the time. They are also incredibly versatile and can be used in so many creative ways.

GOOD FOR
- Constipation and digestive health
- Heart health
- Lowering cholesterol

Constipation and digestive health

Bananas are certainly a dynamo when it comes to digestive health. They are very high in fibre, which will take on many times its own weight in water and swell up. This activates stretch receptors in the gut, which, in turn, stimulates peristalsis – the natural contractions of the gut. This then 'moves everything along'.

Bananas are also rich in a type of very large complex sugar called fructooligosaccharides (FOS). This is a type of sugar that isn't broken down in the usual way sugars are – by enzymes in the saliva and small intestine. They are instead broken down via fermentation by our gut bacteria. When these beneficial bacteria ferment down sugars like FOS, they grow in number and strengthen as a colony. They also secrete by-products, such as something called butyric acid, that stimulate repair mechanisms in the gut wall.

Heart health

Bananas are a great heart-healthy snack, and they have three tricks up their sleeve in that respect. Firstly, bananas are high in the mineral potassium. This mineral is used to regulate the contraction of the heart muscle. It also buffers the mineral sodium. You will have heard a thousand times that we need to reduce salt because the sodium content can raise blood pressure. It does this by slowing down the movement of water through the kidneys' filtration system, which makes us hold on to water. This, in turn, increases the water portion of the blood which creates more pressure against the vessel wall. Sodium also raises blood pressure by causing constriction of the blood vessels, makes them less flexible, which causes the walls to face greater pressure and resistance and the heart to pump. Eating potassium-rich foods means you lose sodium via the urine.

Lowering cholesterol

The second way that bananas can benefit heart health is down to their sterol content. These are fatty substances that are similar in structure to cholesterol but can actually block cholesterol absorption in the gut, resulting in lower serum cholesterol levels over time.

The third way bananas benefit heart health links in well with the second point. They are very rich in soluble fibre. This fibre will also bind to cholesterol in the digestive tract and carry it out of the body via the bowel, which further adds to the lowering of serum cholesterol.

OTHER BENEFITS
Rich in vitamin B6 and manganese

BEST WAY TO EAT
Eaten fresh, use to thicken smoothies, give moisture, sweetness and texture to cakes and baking, and as a base for healthy ice cream

BEETROOT (BEETS)

This is one of my top vegetables and one that has become quite trendy. Roasted, puréed, juiced – they are versatile and true nutrient bombs.

GOOD FOR
- Heart health
- Liver health

Heart health

Beetroot is rich in a group of substances called nitrates. These have been widely studied in recent years in the context of heart health and their influence on the cardiovascular system. Nitrates, once consumed, get converted into nitric oxide, which is produced naturally by the endothelial cells that line the inside of our blood vessels. Nitric oxide causes the smooth muscle that makes up the walls of the blood vessels to relax. When this happens, the vessel widens. As the vessel widens, the pressure against the walls of the vessel reduces. Long story short: increased nitric oxide can transiently lower blood pressure. This same mechanism may also extend some benefit to athletes and exercise enthusiasts because the dilation of blood vessels also leads to an increase in oxygen delivery to the tissues. Greater oxygen delivery equates to greater energy production in tissues. Small-scale studies at Queen Margaret University, Edinburgh, showed that consuming beetroot juice before sporting events was associated with improved performance.

Liver health

Beetroot's intense purple colour pigment – which stains everything it comes into contact with – is delivered by a compound called betacyanin. This substance has, in early studies, been shown to speed up the activity of enzymes in the liver that form part of phase 2 detoxification pathways in the liver involved in disarming harmful substances in the body, ready for removal.

OTHER BENEFITS

High in dietary fibre, which can increase digestive transit time and support gut flora

BEST WAY TO EAT

Juiced, roasted, steamed – this vegetable is versatile

BLUEBERRIES

Blueberries have been true superstars in the health world, and for a while it was as if they were the answer to every conceivable health woe. They earned the coveted 'superfood' title early on, and while that term means absolutely nothing unless you are a marketer, they are a great little ingredient with some notable benefits.

GOOD FOR
- Lowering blood pressure
- Sport and exercise performance, and cognitive function

Lowering blood pressure

Blueberries are very rich in a group of compounds called flavonoids. These are the chemicals that are responsible for the deep purple colour of blueberries. Flavonoids have been very widely studied, and one of the key findings is that they have an influence on our circulatory system. They are taken up by endothelial cells – the cells that make the skin that lines the inner surface of our blood vessels. When they enter endothelial cells, they cause what is thought to be some kind of metabolic distress within the cell that prompts these cells to release a chemical called nitric oxide. This is something they do naturally, but flavonoids ramp up this release considerably. When nitric oxide is released, it causes the smooth muscle that makes up the vessel walls to relax. When these muscle fibres relax, the vessel widens. Because the vessel gets bigger, the pressure exerted against the wall of the vessel by the blood flowing through it is reduced. In short, it lowers blood pressure.

Sport and exercise performance, and cognitive function
The flavonoid response described on the previous page also has an impact on areas such as athletic performance and cognitive function, as it causes an enhanced blood flow. The better the blood flow to tissues, the greater the oxygen saturation of that tissue is, and the more effectively it performs.

OTHER BENEFITS
Rich in vitamin C

BEST WAY TO EAT
Fresh, on porridge, in smoothies

BRAZIL NUTS

These rich and decadent nuts do pack quite the nutritional punch, with one nutrient in particular.

GOOD FOR
- Cellular health

Cellular health

Brazil nuts are one of the few good-quality food sources of the trace element selenium. This vital trace element is a precursor to antioxidant enzymes found within our cells that help to break down and remove waste materials, and also help to protect structures within our cells, particularly DNA from oxidative damage.

OTHER BENEFITS

Rich in copper and magnesium

BEST WAY TO EAT

Eaten raw

BROCCOLI

We are very fortunate that this amazing vegetable grows in such abundance in the Western world. It really is everywhere. But sadly, it is one of those foods that seems to be a real love–hate ingredient. I'm sure if more people really knew how good it is, they would try and eat more of it. It is a great all-rounder on the healthy food scale.

GOOD FOR
- Cellular health

Cellular health

Broccoli, like all cruciferous vegetables, is very rich in a group of compounds called glucosinolates. These are powerfully pungent flavour compounds that deliver heat in ingredients such as mustard, for example. Have you ever bitten into the white core of a cabbage or the central stalk of broccoli and noticed that these taste almost hot? This is the glucosinolates. What is so special about these substances? Well, they have been shown to activate the production of enzymes within our cells that help to keep the cells healthy by disarming harmful substances and protecting DNA from damage. Some claim that this activity may make them an 'anti-cancer food'. Now, that kind of terminology or promise makes me very uneasy indeed, and I think it is inaccurate in some ways. Sure, protecting DNA from damage has an important role to play in protecting against cancer, but this is only in relation to the rest of the environment. If you are smoking heavily, living off pizza, drowning in stress and drinking too much, then a bit of broccoli isn't going to help. But eating more glucosinolate-rich foods is a good idea, just to support the activity of these housekeeping enzymes. Plus, they are rich in many micronutrients right across the board.

OTHER BENEFITS

Rich in magnesium, vitamin C and dietary fibre

BEST WAY TO EAT

Steamed, or my favourite – stir-fried with a little garlic

BROWN RICE

This is one of my favourite grains, full stop. Having spent a great deal of time in Japan, I grew to adore brown rice and it is still very much a staple in my household to this day.

GOOD FOR
- Constipation
- Blood sugar regulation
- Heart health

Constipation

Brown rice is a very high-fibre grain. High-fibre foods will take on several times their own weight in water and swell within the digestive tract. When they do this, they activate stretch receptors in the gut wall, which in turn stimulate a reflexive contraction of the gut wall that moves everything along nicely.

Blood sugar regulation

Refined grains like white rice, white bread, etc. are renowned for causing chaos with our blood sugar levels, sending them soaring and then crashing. However, high-fibre grains like brown rice can have the opposite effect. The high fibre content means that foods like brown rice take much longer to digest and hence take far longer to liberate their sugars. The result is that our blood sugar is drip-fed instead of being carpet-bombed, as is the case with white, refined versions.

Heart health

All high-fibre foods will benefit cardiovascular health to one extent or another. This is because the fibre will bind to cholesterol in the gut and carry it away, lowering serum concentrations of cholesterol. There is also a compound found in brown rice called gamma-oryzanol, which several studies have shown can lower LDL cholesterol (see page 83).

OTHER BENEFITS

Rich in B vitamins

BEST WAY TO EAT

Risottos, to thicken soups, in salads, as a staple grain side dish

BULGUR WHEAT

I love bulgur wheat. It has a delicious nutty flavour, and is super filling and nutrient rich.

> **GOOD FOR**
> - Sustained energy
> - Digestive health
> - Heart health

Sustained energy

Bulgur wheat can help give us sustained energy for two reasons. Firstly, it is a very slow-release carbohydrate source. The slowness is because of the high level of fibre, which causes bulgur wheat to be digested much more slowly than something like white rice. This slow digestion drip-feeds our blood sugar, which, in turn, gives us a sustained energy level without all the peaks and troughs.

The second reason why bulgur wheat can be a great energy food is because it is so rich in B vitamins. These nutrients are used to turn glucose into adenosine triphosphate (ATP) – the energy source our cells use.

Digestive health

Bulgur wheat, like all high-fibre foods, supports digestion by swelling up and stimulating the rhythmical contractions of the digestive system that move things along.

Heart health

High-fibre foods support cardiovascular health by binding to cholesterol in the gut and carrying it away, which has been clinically proven to lower serum cholesterol.

OTHER BENEFITS

Rich in magnesium and iron

BEST WAY TO EAT

In soups, as a rice alternative in risottos (barlotto),
to make tabouleh

BUTTERNUT SQUASH

I adore these vegetables, particularly during the winter months.
They are sweet, full of flavour and versatile.

GOOD FOR
- Skin health
- Heart health

Skin health

Butternut squash is a great source of fat-soluble antioxidants,
particularly beta carotene. This is the substance that gives the
squash its vivid orange colour. Beta carotene, as a fat-soluble
antioxidant, can accumulate in the fatty subcutaneous layer
of the skin. When it accumulates here, it can offer localized
antioxidant protection to important structures that are housed
in this fatty layer, such as collagen and elastin fibres that give
skin its structural integrity, and also the pilosebaceous unit –
the area where the sebaceous gland and hair follicle meet.
This localized protection can help to reduce daily oxidative
damage that can lead to accelerated ageing of the skin.
Fat-soluble antioxidants such as beta carotene can also deliver
some anti-inflammatory activity, and their regular consumption
may be of benefit to sufferers of eczema and acne.

Heart health

The carotenoid group of antioxidants can help to prevent
oxidation of fatty substances whereby chemicals, cells and
tissues can become damaged by unstable molecules that
are missing an oxygen atom and need to find one at all costs,
causing untold damage in the process.

One such substance in our circulation is cholesterol.
Cholesterol is supposed to be there, and is an important

substance in the body. However, certain lifestyle factors can increase our susceptibility to this cholesterol oxidizing, which can cause damage to blood vessel walls and kick-start the process of heart disease – the formation of plaque within the vessel walls. By reducing this oxidation, antioxidants like beta carotene and vitamin E, for instance, can offer long-term protection against heart disease.

OTHER BENEFITS
High in vitamin C and dietary fibre

BEST WAY TO EAT
Roasted, in soups, grated raw in salads; even works well in a juice

CABBAGE

Cabbage is one of the best foods that grow abundantly in many parts of the world, but the way so many people cook it makes it another of the unpopular ones. Boiling it to death and creating a stink bomb is not the way to get the best out of this beautiful family of ingredients.

GOOD FOR
- Cellular health
- Heart health

Cellular health

Cabbages, like broccoli – see page 135 – are very rich in the compound isothiocyanate, which has been shown to increase the production and activity of key enzymes that our cells use to disarm harmful substances within them, remove waste materials from cells more effectively and protect our DNA from damage. Keeping cells healthy is vital as we get older, and supporting these natural processes helps us immensely in this respect.

Heart health

Cabbages can benefit heart health in several ways. Firstly, there are specific phytochemical compounds that have been shown to reduce the levels of homocysteine – a substance that has been associated with increased risk of heart disease.

The real hero in terms of heart health, however, is the red cabbage. This is due to the purple colour pigment that is created by a group of compounds called flavonoids. These widely studied substances stimulate the release of a chemical called nitric oxide from the inner lining of our blood vessels. Nitric oxide causes the muscle fibres that make up the blood vessel walls to relax, which makes the vessels bigger and reduces the pressure within them. Nitric oxide also helps to protect the inner lining of vessels from damage.

OTHER BENEFITS

High levels of vitamin C, high dietary fibre, B vitamins

BEST WAY TO EAT

Lightly steamed, sautéed with garlic

CANNELLINI BEANS

These are one of my favourite beans that make their way into all manner of dishes, from Italian stews to Indian curries.

GOOD FOR
- Digestive health
- Skin health

Digestive health

The high fibre content of cannellini beans provides two major benefits for the health of the digestive system. Firstly, fibre will swell up within the gut by absorbing water, which stimulates the normal contractions in the gut that move things along. Secondly, some of the fibres in the beans will be untouched by digestive enzymes higher up in the digestive tract, and instead are broken down by the bacteria that live in the gut via fermentation. When this fermentation breakdown occurs, the bacterial colony begins to increase in numbers. Also during this fermentation process, by-products are released that help to repair and maintain the inner surfaces of the gut.

Skin health

Cannellini beans can benefit the health of the skin in two ways. The first is through their rich source of zinc, a mineral used by the sebaceous glands in the skin to regulate oil secretions. If skin is too oily or too dry, adequate zinc in the diet can even things out. Zinc is also used by our white blood cells to code genes that regulate the way in which white cells respond to pathogens, so in issues such as acne, where there is active infection, it can speed up healing time.

The second way that cannellini beans can help the skin is in offering some protection against sun damage. This is thanks to a substance called ferulic acid, which can actually enhance the effects of other key antioxidants that protect the skin, such as vitamin E and carotenoids.

OTHER BENEFITS

Rich in B vitamins and magnesium

BEST WAY TO EAT

In hummus, stews, curries

CARROTS

This wonderful vegetable is as cheap as it comes and is super versatile. Carrots may seem very dull and 'everyday', but they pack quite the nutritional punch.

GOOD FOR
- Skin health
- Healthy eyes
- Heart health

Skin health

Carrots are an amazing skin food. This is thanks to their massive levels of beta carotene, the antioxidant substance responsible for their bright orange colour. This fat-soluble antioxidant – as we found out with Butternut Squash on page 141 – can begin to accumulate in the fatty subcutaneous layer of the skin that houses important structures such as the collagen and elastin fibre matrix that gives skin its structural integrity, suppleness and flexibility. The subcutaneous layer of the skin also houses the pilosebaceous unit, where the hair follicle and sebaceous gland meet. By accumulating in the subcutaneous layer, fat-soluble antioxidants such as carotenoids offer localized protection to these structures from free radical damage.

Healthy eyes

They say that carrots help you to see in the dark. Beta carotene is the plant source of vitamin A. It is actually two vitamin A units bound together head to head, which the body cleaves in two when vitamin A is required. Vitamin A protects the health of the cornea and guards against macular degeneration, the oxidative damage to the macula (the central part of the retina at the back of the eye) that can lead to vision loss.

Heart health

Beta carotene as an antioxidant can reduce oxidation of lipids (fatty substances) and lipid-derived substances, which means it can reduce oxidation of cholesterol (where cholesterol reacts with oxygen and can potentially become toxic), a reaction that can cause significant damage to the walls of blood vessels. This, in turn, can trigger the cascade of events that eventually leads to plaque formation and heart disease. Beta carotene can also deliver some anti-inflammatory benefit locally, even though it doesn't remain in circulation for very long.

OTHER BENEFITS

Rich in vitamins C and K and potassium

BEST WAY TO EAT

Juiced, eaten raw with salads or dipped in hummus

CASHEW NUTS

I adore these. They are rich, creamy and can be a great base for sauces and sweets.

GOOD FOR
- Vegan calcium source
- Cardiovascular health

Vegan calcium source

Calcium is a diversely distributed mineral for which we seem to have a deep running fear of not ingesting enough, especially those adopting a vegan diet. Cashews are a rich source of easy-to-absorb calcium.

Cardiovascular health

Like all nuts, cashews are a great food for the health of the cardiovascular system, and this is due to the fats and fat-derived substances in them. They are rich sources of polyunsaturated fatty acids that can offer benefit to heart health by means of improving the LDL/HDL cholesterol ratios (see page 83). As mentioned in relation to other nuts, cashew nuts are rich in vitamin E, which is an antioxidant with a specific affinity for fats. It helps to reduce the oxidation of cholesterol (see opposite), a process that can damage the blood vessels and set the stage for cardiovascular disease.

BEST WAY TO EAT

Ideally eaten raw; heating and cooking can damage the delicate fats they contain

CELERY

Celery is one of those salad staples that is overlooked in other dishes because no one ever knows what to do with it! I have to be honest; it isn't my favourite food in the world, but it is interesting from a nutritional point of view.

GOOD FOR
- Pain reduction
- Urinary health

Pain reduction

Celery may be the furthest thing from your mind when it comes to pain reduction, but there is a compound in celery called 3-N-butylphthalide (3NB for short) that has been shown to have analgaesic qualities. The exact mechanisms of action are yet to be determined, but it's interesting nonetheless.

Urinary health

Celery acts as a diuretic. Any fan of juicing will know that a celery-laden juice will have you peeing profusely! This is due to two elements. The first element is a group of chemicals called coumarins, part of the chemistry that gives celery its distinctive smell. In the herbal medicine world, coumarins have been known to increase urinary output. The second element is the high level of potassium. This mineral increases the movement of fluid through the nephron – the filtration system of the kidney.

OTHER BENEFITS
Rich in B vitamins, copper, vitamin K, folate and carotenoids

BEST WAY TO EAT
Juiced or eaten raw

CHICKPEAS (GARBANZO BEANS)

These have become a staple in the health-food world over the years and I'm a big fan.

GOOD FOR
- Appetite management
- Heart health

Appetite management

Chickpeas are a great food for increasing satiety. This is all thanks to their very high fibre content. Fibre has long been associated with controlling appetite, as it physically stretches the upper digestive tract and stimulates the release of hormones that shut off appetite. Chickpeas are over 20% fibre!

Heart health

Like all high-fibre foods, there will be considerable benefits for the health of the heart. This is because the fibre binds to cholesterol and carries it out via the bowel. This, in turn, lowers serum cholesterol, as the body mobilizes it back to the liver where it is used in the manufacture of bile acids.

OTHER BENEFITS
Rich in zinc and B vitamins

BEST WAY TO EAT
In hummus, salads, curries

COCOA/CACAO

It's official. Chocolate is good for you. Okay, I will backtrack a little and say cacao, the unrefined, un-sugared dried ground cocoa bean is very good for you! Not only is it a taste of heaven, it has an incredibly complex biochemistry and nutritional profile.

GOOD FOR
- Cardiovascular health
- Mind and mood
- Natural energy boost

Cardiovascular health

Cocoa is packed to the hilt with a group of compounds called flavonoids. These compounds have been very widely researched and are known to cause the cells that line our blood vessels to release high levels of a compound called nitric oxide, which induces the muscles in the blood vessel walls to relax. When they relax, the blood vessel widens, which lowers the pressure within it. Cacao is also very high in the mineral magnesium, which also encourages relaxation of the smooth muscles in blood vessel walls.

Mind and mood

Raw cacao is rich in two powerful compounds that have a very interesting effect upon the mind and mood. The first is a substance called anandamide, which is also naturally produced in our brain. It enhances motivation and pleasure, and is said to give feelings of bliss. The next compound is something called phenylethylamine (PEA for short), which is a powerful mood elevator. It is also present in regular chocolate and cocoa but at much lower concentrations. It is a compound that is quite rapidly broken down, by an enzyme called monoamine oxidase, before it gets the chance to reach the brain. However, the high concentration in raw cacao does allow a small amount to get through and have neurological effects, all be they mild.

Natural energy boost

Cocoa does contain a stimulant compound called theobromine, which is a close cousin to caffeine. It is a stimulant, but it seems to have less of a 'burn-out' after-effect than caffeine. I would still advise not overconsuming it, though.

BEST WAY TO EAT

In smoothies, in dips or a good 80% cocoa solids chocolate bar

COCONUT

Coconut products have become an absolute monster sector of the health-food industry. The world has gone coconut mad! Some…well…most of the claims made about it are daft at best and dangerous at worst. There has been much debate around the saturated fat issue, which still appears to have not been adequately answered, and there are a lot of grey areas surrounding it, that's for sure.

GOOD FOR
- Resilient fat source
- Antiviral

Resilient fat source

Coconut oil is one of the best choices of high-temperature cooking fats because it can be heated to very high temperatures without forming trans fats, one of the most harmful substances that arises from frying foods, and which has been linked to heart disease and unhealthy cholesterol levels. While I wouldn't recommend using coconut oil for all of your cooking, for the high-temperature work it is definitely a winner.

Antiviral

One of the main fats found in coconut oil is a substance called lauric acid, which has been shown to have some interesting antiviral properties. It actually blocks the way viruses enter our cells and multiply.

BEST WAY TO EAT
Use as a cooking oil for high-temperature work only

CRANBERRIES

Cranberries only really seem to appear at one time of year – Christmas. Finding them fresh in the supermarket at any other time is a challenge, which is a shame, as they have a great antioxidant content. Like all berries, they contain significant amounts of vitamin C, and are rich in flavonoids, which deliver their well-known cardiovascular benefits (see page 133). Cranberries have a couple of potential additional benefits, too.

GOOD FOR
- Urinary health

Urinary health

Possibly the most well-known health benefit of cranberries is in the context of UTI treatment. This reputation is partially deserved, and some studies support this, while other studies have found little benefit. It seems it all comes down to the bacteria that is causing the infection in the first place. When the UTI is a simple one caused by *E. coli,* the polyphenols in cranberry can reduce the capacity of this bacteria to adhere to the inner walls of the urinary tract, making it less able to trigger the immunological response that delivers the symptoms associated with a UTI. There are also substances in cranberry, like ursolic acid, that seem to influence inflammatory pathways to some degree and may offer an additional degree of support.

OTHER BENEFITS

Very high in vitamin C; high levels of flavonoids make cranberries, like all berries, a beneficial ingredient to support heart health

BEST WAY TO EAT

Juiced, eaten fresh as a sharp, sour twist in a fruit salad

DATES

Dates have achieved almost cult status in the health world in recent years. The array of crazy desserts and concoctions based on them is really quite incredible. It is worth bearing in mind that they are very sugar dense, so just because they do deliver some nutrients and have some potentially beneficial properties, they shouldn't be eaten with reckless abandon.

GOOD FOR
→ Digestive health

Digestive health

Dates are incredibly high in dietary fibre. This means they take on many times their own weight in water, swell up and stimulate peristalsis, natural contractions, in the gut, helping to 'move everything along'. The fibre in dates can also benefit the health of the good bacteria that live in the gut.

OTHER BENEFITS

Rich in iron, magnesium, manganese and vitamin B6

BEST WAY TO EAT

Eaten whole, baked into healthy desserts or dipped in peanut butter for a heavenly snack

FENNEL

The distinctive aniseed flavour of fennel is a quite divisive, but its versatility makes it a kitchen hero for me.

GOOD FOR
- Digestive health

Digestive health

Fennel has been a remedy for indigestion and bloating for decades, all due to the essential oils it contains, which also give it its aniseed flavour. These volatile oils can relax the gut wall and disperse gas, easing bloating and distention.

OTHER BENEFITS

High in dietary fibre, vitamin C and calcium

BEST WAY TO EAT

Juiced, roasted, puréed

FLAXSEEDS (LINSEEDS)

Flaxseeds (also known as linseeds) are one of those staples that have been on the health-food store shelves for decades. Being such a staple, there have been some really weird and wonderful claims made around them, some of which are rather far-fetched. They are a nutritious ingredient and have some very well-documented health benefits, and are something I eat very regularly, several times a week.

GOOD FOR
- Cardiovascular health
- Digestive health
- Powerful antioxidant source

Cardiovascular health

One important thing about flaxseeds is that when they get wet they become gooey and gel-like – they take on many times their own weight in water and create a gelatinous paste. This is key to both their cardiovascular health- and digestive health-supporting properties, and this action of taking on water and forming a gel happens in the gut. In the context of heart health, this gel-like substance that forms can actually trap cholesterol that is in the gut, bind to it to prevent it from being absorbed and then remove it from the body via the bowel. This is cholesterol that is both dietary in origin and has arrived in the gut from the liver during digestion, and the process of flaxseed gel binding to it and removing it ultimately leads to lowered serum cholesterol.

Digestive health

Flaxseeds benefit digestive health again by the swelling and gel formation that occurs in the gut. This will, as expected, naturally cause gut contents to expand and bulk out, which, in turn, stimulates stretch receptors in the gut wall. As soon as these receptors are stimulated, there is a responding contraction of the gut wall, known as peristalsis, and this keeps gut contents moving along, ensuring we are 'regular'.

By keeping gut contents moving, we also create an environment that is favourable for a healthy diverse colony of bacteria to grow and flourish.

Powerful antioxidant source

Flaxseeds are a rich source of a group of substances called lignans. These compounds have a potent antioxidant activity, and they also appear to deliver cardiovascular benefits by means of reducing blood pressure. One note here, though: the seeds will need to be crushed to liberate the lignans.

BEST WAY TO EAT

Crushed and sprinkled on cereals, stews, etc.

GARLIC

Garlic seems to make its way into almost every savoury dish that I prepare. It gives a beautiful base richness and is nutritious, too.

GOOD FOR
- Heart and circulation
- Colds and flu
- Inflammatory conditions

Heart and circulation

Garlic contains a potent compound known as ajoene, which interacts with something called the platelet aggregation factor, a compound that regulates the rate and extent to which blood clots. Some surgeons and dentists even advise patients against eating garlic shortly before surgery in case it increases bleeding. On a day-to-day basis, however, it can reduce the risk of clotting, making it helpful against strokes and heart attacks.

Colds and flu

Garlic contains a group of powerful essential oils that can only be removed from the body through the breath, rather than the usual routes of elimination through the bowels and urine. As we breathe out, they move through the respiratory tract and can kill off bugs and viruses, such as those that can cause colds and flu.

Inflammatory conditions

Raw garlic is actually a reasonably effective anti-inflammatory due to a compound called diallyl disulphide. This compound breaks down drastically on cooking, though.

BEST WAY TO EAT
Eaten raw or lightly cooked

GINGER

Ginger has a stunning flavour and it adds real zing and life to Asian and fusion dishes. For centuries, it has traditionally also been used as a medicine in many cultures.

GOOD FOR
- Inflammatory conditions
- Nausea

Inflammatory conditions

Ginger is one of the most powerful anti-inflammatories there is. The strong, spicy essential oils that give it its lively flavour have been shown by thousands of studies to interrupt certain aspects of the chemical reaction that occurs when inflammation is triggered.

Nausea

Ginger has a long-standing reputation as a useful remedy for the treatment of mild nausea, from morning sickness to motion sickness. It isn't clear how it does this, but many people believe it works by stimulating the production of digestive juices.

BEST WAY TO EAT
Eaten raw, lightly sautéed, crystallized (candied)

GRAPEFRUIT

Grapefruit used to be the staple dieter's breakfast. I remember eating half a pink grapefruit every day as a kid and adoring it. There were all manner of tall tales surrounding it back in the 1980s – it was hailed as a miraculous fat-burning fruit. While this is rather improbable, it is a wonderfully healthy ingredient.

GOOD FOR
- Antioxidant intake
- Cellular health

Antioxidant intake

Pink and red grapefruit get their colour from carotenoid compounds such as lycopene. Increased intakes of lycopene from foods like (bell peppers, tomatoes, pink grapefruit, etc. have been linked to reduced risk of prostate issues.

Cellular health

Phytochemicals in grapefruit called limonoids have been shown to increase the formation of glutathione-S-transferase, an enzyme that is involved in making harmful substances and waste products more water soluble so that they can be easily excreted from the body.

OTHER BENEFITS

High pectin content means that there can be some degree of cholesterol reduction (see pages 119 and 182 for apples and pears for more details on pectin); high vitamin C content

BEST WAY TO EAT

Eaten fresh or juiced

GRAPES

Grapes have been widely linked with health, from the stereotypical bag of grapes taken to people in hospital, through to the old adage of a glass of red wine a day helping the heart. Some of this association is certainly justified.

> **GOOD FOR**
> ‣ Heart health
> ‣ Cellular health

Heart health

Red and black grapes and red wine have long been associated with heart health, and studies support this. They benefit heart health in two ways. The substances in the grapes that give them their deep purple colour that extends into red wine are called flavonoids. These compounds have been widely researched and found to have interesting effects on our circulation. They get taken up by the endothelial cells that line the inside of blood vessels and cause them to secrete nitric oxide. When this happens, the nitric oxide moves into the muscle tissue that makes up the vessel walls and causes the fibres to relax. As they relax, the vessel widens and the pressure within it reduces. Consequently, these substances lower blood pressure.

The release of nitric oxide also protects the endothelium from damage that can occur when cholesterol oxidizes – a reaction that can trigger the first stages of heart disease. There is also some evidence to show that flavonoids can improve LDL/HDL cholesterol ratios (see page 83).

Cellular health

Another substance in grapes and wine is probably the most famous. Called resveratrol, this substance has been shown to activate certain genes associated with longevity called sirtuins. These genes are also associated with reduced cellular damage, and accelerated fat burning.

OTHER BENEFITS
Vitamin C, antioxidant, anti-inflammatory

BEST WAY TO EAT
Grapes eaten fresh; glass of red wine with dinner

JERUSALEM ARTICHOKES (SUNCHOKES)

These funny, knobbly roots are a superhero food in my eyes. Weirdly, though, they aren't artichokes, and nobody can find any kind of association with Jerusalem.

GOOD FOR
- Gut flora support

Gut flora support

Jerusalem artichokes have gained something of a bad reputation – some people can experience noticeable bloating and gas after eating them. But as unpleasant as this can be for susceptible individuals, it is a sign of them working their magic. Jerusalem artichokes are very rich in a special type of large molecular weight sugar called a polysaccharide, specifically inulin.

Some polysaccharides can be broken down in the gut like other carbohydrates. Others, like inulin, can only be broken down via fermentation by gut bacteria. When this happens, we can feel bloated and as if warfare is going on in the gut. However, when our gut flora feeds on these sugars to break them down, they start to reproduce in number, grow and flourish, strengthening the bacterial colony. Also, as the gut flora break these sugars down, other substances such as butyrate are released as a by-product, which can stimulate the repair and maintenance of the gut.

OTHER BENEFITS
High in fibre

BEST WAY TO EAT
Roasted or used in soups

KALE

You can't go anywhere without seeing kale in a healthy recipe or plastered all over social media. It is fair to say that some of the weird and wonderful claims written about it are a bit far-fetched, but it is a great, nutritious green vegetable.

GOOD FOR
- Bone health

Bone health

Kale is a great source of minerals that are vital to the health of the skeleton. For decades we have been told that dairy products are the number one source of calcium. Sure, they are an important source, but not the only one. Not everyone can consume dairy, and many people choose not to, so it is reassuring to know there are alternatives. Kale is rich in a whole cocktail of minerals important to the health of the bones, including calcium, magnesium and phosphorous.

OTHER BENEFITS

Vitamins C and K and dietary fibre

BEST WAY TO EAT

Lightly steamed, used in a sauce or even eaten raw; DO NOT boil it to death

LEEKS

Leeks are one of my favourite ingredients for building flavour; sweet, aromatic, just lovely.

GOOD FOR
- Digestive health

Digestive health

Leeks, like all of the allium family, are very rich in the prebiotic sugar inulin. This is a very large, complex sugar that requires fermentation by our gut bacteria to be broken down. When this happens, the bacterial colony starts to increase in number. When fermenting inulin, the gut flora also produce short-chain fatty acids (SCFAs) as a by-product, which help to repair and maintain the gut lining.

OTHER BENEFITS
High in fibre, iron and folate

BEST WAY TO EAT
Sautéed as a flavour base in savoury dishes; also griddled and roasted

LEMONS AND LIMES

Lemons and limes are two of the powerhouse citrus fruits. They were, in fact, the fruits that kept us healthy on the high seas, earning us Brits the nickname 'Limeys'. So what makes these seemingly ordinary fruits so special?

GOOD FOR
- Antibiotic activity
- Cardiovascular health

Antibiotic activity

This may sound slightly implausible, but a group of compounds – in limes in particular – called flavanol glycosides has been shown to deliver antibiotic activities. In some trials in West Africa, for example, the inclusion of lime juice in meals proved effective at reducing cholera incidence.

Cardiovascular health

Lemons and limes are both very rich in potent flavonoids, similar to the ones we have described several times (see pages 132 and 163 for blueberries and grapes). Citrus bioflavonoids seem to protect smaller weaker blood vessels like capillaries from damage. They make the fragile walls of these vessels more resilient to damage from normal day-to-day metabolic events.

OTHER BENEFITS
Rich in vitamin C and folate

BEST WAY TO EAT
Juiced

LENTILS

Lentils are a great tool for everything, from thickening dishes to adding an additional protein hit to dishes.

GOOD FOR
- Heart health
- Plant-based protein

Heart health

As is the case with many high-fibre foods, they will support the health of the heart by binding to cholesterol in the digestive system and carrying it away. This is cholesterol that has left the liver during fat digestion that will get reabsorbed later on in the digestive tract, where it will then be put to use elsewhere. If we head this cholesterol off at the pass, then cholesterol that is in circulation will be sent to the liver to be used for digestive purposes. This, in turn, lowers the serum concentrations of cholesterol. Red lentils in particular are very rich in these types of fibres.

Plant-based protein

Although it is incredibly difficult not to get enough protein, even as a strict vegan some people will want to get more – athletes, for example. If this is you, then lentils can be one of your best friends, as they are over 37% protein. That's pretty impressive for a plant-based food.

OTHER BENEFITS
Rich in B vitamins and iron

BEST WAY TO EAT
Stewed; in soups, dips and purées

MACKEREL

This wonderful oily fish has a strong flavour that puts some people off, while others absolutely love it. Mackerel is great in a multitude of dishes and it's super easy to prepare.

GOOD FOR
- Inflammatory conditions
- Heart and circulation
- Osteoporosis and rickets

Inflammatory conditions

Mackerel is incredibly high in vital omega-3 fatty acids, and these help the body to produce its own in-built anti-inflammatory compounds. This makes mackerel, like all oily fish, great for inflammatory conditions.

Heart and circulation

The omega-3 fatty acids have a very favourable effect upon cholesterol levels, and can also protect blood vessel walls from inflammatory damage.

Osteoporosis and rickets

Oily fish, especially mackerel, is very high in vitamin D, which is vital for the proper utilization of calcium in the body. The main source of vitamin D for humans is the conversion of cholesterol into vitamin D upon exposure to ultraviolet radiation (UV rays) – in other words, the sun! Thankfully, there are also a few food sources, and oily fish and lean dairy products are top of the list.

BEST WAY TO EAT
Grilled with crushed beetroot (beets) and horseradish;
hot smoked with a salad

MANGOES

One of my all-time favourite fruits, hands down. Sweet, sumptuous and antioxidant rich. What's not to love?

GOOD FOR
➤ Skin health

Skin health

Mangoes are packed with an antioxidant substance called beta carotene, which is what makes them orange, and is also found in carrots, sweet potatoes, etc. This is a vital nutrient for healthy skin. People often talk about antioxidants for skin health, and just kind of lump them all together and assume that if it has antioxidants, then it is good for the skin and that's the end of it. This is inaccurate thinking, as the actions of antioxidants vary wildly. That being said, antioxidants can be divided into two distinct groups – water soluble and fat soluble. Water-soluble antioxidants like vitamin C are active in our general circulation for a limited amount of time, then are metabolized and excreted from the body. Fat-soluble antioxidants, on the other hand, don't stay in circulation very long. By their very nature they want to move out of circulation and migrate into fatty tissues. Second to the brain, the most abundant fatty tissue in the body is the subcutaneous layer of the skin. This layer houses important structures such as collagen and elastin fibres that give skin its structural support. These structures are susceptible to oxidative damage. With a good intake of fat-soluble antioxidants, like the carotenoids found in mangoes, they can begin to accumulate in the subcutaneous layer, and offer localized antioxidant protection for these important structures. The short story is that these compounds can offer anti-ageing support for the skin when consumed regularly.

OTHER BENEFITS

Great source of vitamin C and high in fibre

BEST WAY TO EAT

Fresh, or frozen and then puréed into a sorbet

MILK AND DAIRY

This is a contentious area of nutrition. I personally don't take dairy milk, but I do have feta or goat's cheese now and again. For the purposes of this chapter, let's have a look at what dairy can provide, although it's worth noting that this can be obtained from other sources, too.

GOOD FOR
- Skeletal health
- Rich vitamin A source

Skeletal health

This actually has very little to do with calcium, because calcium is a very commonly distributed mineral, found in many foods. Dairy does, however, have good levels of vitamin D, which is responsible for increasing calcium absorption from the digestive tract. It is also responsible for moving calcium between the skeleton and the bloodstream, and this is a two-way traffic flow. If blood levels go up following ingestion of a calcium-rich meal, then vitamin D will transport excess to the skeleton where it is laid down. Likewise, if blood calcium levels drop for long enough, vitamin D will facilitate the liberation of calcium from the skeleton and send it into circulation. Vitamin D also regulates bone remodelling and ensures bone hardness.

Rich vitamin A source

Dairy products are a rich source of vitamin A in the retinol form, vital for healthy eyes, mucous membranes and immune system.

BEST WAY TO EAT

In general, fermented dairy, such as yogurt and cheese, tends to be better tolerated

MUSHROOMS

Mushrooms are a bit of a mixed bag nutritionally. Some are rather benign, while others can have some incredible benefits for the body. Most everyday mushrooms will be good sources of some B vitamins, and certain varieties of chestnut mushrooms will be grown in an environment that allows them to be rich in vitamin D. However, the ones that are really the powerhouses for me are the shiitake mushrooms, so the benefits listed below are for those.

GOOD FOR
- Immune system health
- Heart and circulation

Immune system health

Shiitake mushrooms are one of the few varieties of mushrooms that contain a very powerful, unique sugar called a polysaccharide. There are many of these in nature, but the type found in shiitake is beta glucans, and these have been researched globally for over 40 years. One area in which there is the strongest evidence is the effect they have upon the immune system. They have been shown to cause an increase in the production of white blood cells (our immune system's army), and their response to pathogens or damaged cells. Just a small amount of these compounds daily can really give the immune system a bit of a kick.

Heart and circulation

A decade or two ago, a substance in shiitake mushrooms called eritadenine was discovered. It was found that this compound could lower 'bad' (LDL) cholesterol, while improving levels of 'good' (HDL) cholesterol (see page 83). It is believed that it does this by influencing the way in which the liver produces cholesterol in the first place.

BEST WAY TO EAT

Lightly cooked is best, as some people can have issues with raw shiitake mushrooms

OATS

Oats have been the staple of healthy eaters for decades, and rightfully so.

GOOD FOR
- Healthy nervous system
- Heart health

Healthy nervous system

Oats have been used in Western herbal medicine for centuries as a supportive remedy for the nervous system, delivering a calming and soothing activity for nervous exhaustion. As a medical herbalist myself, I can certainly report, anecdotally at least, that this can be the case. The active constituents responsible here aren't fully established, but oats are very rich in B vitamins, which are responsible for many functions within the nervous system, such as the manufacture of neurotransmitters.

Heart health

Oats contain unique types of soluble fibre called beta glucans that have been widely clinically researched and proven to lower cholesterol.

OTHER BENEFITS
Rich in B vitamins, zinc and magnesium

BEST WAY TO EAT
Porridge or oat bars

OLIVES

I absolutely adore olives. A bowlful in the late afternoon while on holiday, ideally overlooking the sea … bliss!! The beauty is, these little morsels are incredibly good for us, too.

GOOD FOR
- Digestive health
- Heart and circulation

Digestive health

One of the most noticeable things about olives is their bitter flavour, and this is key to how they can help digestion. When we taste something bitter, a nervous reflex takes place, and as a result of this, the gall bladder contracts and releases a squirt of bile. Bile is essential for fat digestion, and also works as the body's own built-in laxative. This same reflex also increases the production of gastric juices, so protein digestion will be improved slightly.

Heart and circulation

The fatty acids in olive oil, primarily the omega-9 family of fatty acids, have been shown on many occasions to be beneficial for the health of the heart. They can increase the levels of 'good' (HDL) cholesterol, and decrease the 'bad' (LDL) cholesterol (see page 83). Oleic acid in olive oil also seems to have a beneficial effect on blood pressure.

BEST WAY TO EAT
Eaten whole, or extra virgin olive oil used on salads or for dipping

ONIONS

Onions, particularly the red variety, feature in almost every savoury dish that I cook. They are key to building deep flavour, and their health benefits are great.

GOOD FOR
- Digestive health
- Heart health

Digestive health

Just as with leeks, all types of onion are very rich in the prebiotic inulin that builds and strengthens our bacterial colony.

Heart health

Red onions are particularly beneficial for heart health, all because of the purple colour pigment. This comes from the group of phytochemicals known as flavonoids. These substances have been widely studied, with a great deal of the work being done in the UK at the University of Reading, and shown to be absorbed by the endothelial cells that line the inside of our blood vessels. When these cells absorb flavonoids, there is a reflex metabolic distress that causes endothelial cells to secrete nitric oxide, a substance that prompts blood vessels to widen, lowering the pressure within them. Nitric oxide also protects the endothelium from the type of damage that triggers heart disease.

OTHER BENEFITS
High in sulphur, vitamin C and folic acid

BEST WAY TO EAT
Sautéed with garlic as a flavour base or eaten raw in salads

ORANGES

Oranges are one of the most widely consumed fruits in the world. This is mostly due to the global popularity of orange juice. Most people associate oranges and their healthy rating with their vitamin C content. This, however, isn't as high as has been played. Sure, there's a fair bit in there, but spinach, for example, contains far more gram for gram. Oranges have quite a complex phytochemistry, and this is where their biggest benefits arise from.

GOOD FOR
- Heart health
- Cellular health

Heart health

Oranges can play several important roles in supporting heart health. This is mostly thanks to the presence of a type of flavanone called hesperidin. This substance has, in experimental models at least, been shown to lower cholesterol and improve LDL/HDL ratios (see page 83). Hesperidin has also been shown to reduce blood pressure. There are other flavonoid compounds present in oranges that take this a step further. Flavonoids have been widely studied in the UK and have been shown to lower blood pressure by causing the cells that line the inside of the blood vessels to release something called nitric oxide prompting the muscular walls of the vessels to relax, thus lowering the pressure within them.

Cellular health

Oranges are a great source of citrus-specific phytochemicals called limonoids. These substances have been shown to have antimutagenic activity, which means they can help protect genetic material in cells from damage that can trigger changes in cells that potentially lead to cancer.

OTHER BENEFITS

Oranges do, of course, have a reasonable vitamin C content and are also a great fibre source when eaten whole (i.e. in whole segments rather than juiced).

BEST WAY TO EAT

Eaten whole or juiced; however, if you go for the juice, make sure that it is freshly squeezed – juice from concentrate has had most of the good stuff blasted out of it during processing

PARSNIPS

I really love parsnips, especially roasted with a Sunday lunch. Gorgeous!

GOOD FOR
- Digestive health

Digestive health

Parsnips benefit digestive health in two ways. Firstly, they are very high in dietary fibre, which takes on many times its own weight in water, adding bulk to the gut contents and stimulating the movement of food through the digestive system. The other way parsnips offer benefit is in their content of fructooligosaccharide (FOS), a large polysaccharide that feeds gut bacteria, similar to what we see with Jerusalem artichokes (sunchokes) and leeks (see pages 165 and 167).

OTHER BENEFITS
High in folate and manganese

BEST WAY TO EAT
Roasted, made into purées and soups

PEARS

Another popular fruit, which I love to eat with blue cheese.

GOOD FOR
- Digestive health
- Cardiovascular health

Digestive health

Pears are a great source of the soluble fibre pectin. Those of you who are jam makers may well be familiar with this. Pectin has two big benefits. Firstly, as a fibre, it takes on many times its own weight in water and swells up. When it swells, it activates stretch receptors in the gut, which stimulates the natural contractions in the gut wall that move everything along, keeping us 'regular'. This fibre also supports the growth and stability of gut flora – the bacterial colony that lives in the gut and regulates virtually every aspect of digestive health.

Cardiovascular health

The second big benefit of pectin is in cardiovascular health. When it takes on water and swells in the gut, it forms a gel-like substance. This traps cholesterol that is in the gut and that has come from the liver during digestion, and prevents it being reabsorbed. This has the knock-on effect of lowering serum cholesterol levels.

OTHER BENEFITS
High in vitamin C

BEST WAY TO EAT
Eaten fresh or puréed

PEPPERS (BELL PEPPERS)

I eat peppers almost every day, often in my lunchtime salad.

GOOD FOR
- Skin health
- Heart health

Skin health

Peppers contain several nutrients that can benefit skin health. Firstly, similar to many orange foods, they are rich in fat-soluble antioxidants such as carotenoids. These accumulate in the subcutaneous layer of the skin and protect collagen and elastin from damage, delivering an anti-ageing effect.

Peppers are also rich in vitamin C, vital in manufacturing collagen. The more effectively we make collagen, the more protection we have against premature ageing and sagging skin.

Finally, peppers contain the mineral silica, responsible for the shine on a pepper's outer skin. Silica helps strengthen the extra cellular matrix, a lattice that holds cells in place. Keeping this matrix healthy can keep the skin looking smooth and firm.

Heart health

Peppers are rich in carotenoids. These fat-soluble antioxidants have a particular affinity for disarming lipid-derived oxidative substances. They can help to reduce cholesterol oxidation, a process that can damage the inner surface of our blood vessels.

OTHER BENEFITS
Rich in magnesium, thiamin, folate and potassium

BEST WAY TO EAT
Eaten raw as a crudité or in salads; in ratatouille and soups

PINEAPPLES

Pineapples are one of my favourite fruits. Zingy and fragrant. What's not to love?

GOOD FOR
- Anti-inflammatory boost
- Digestive health

Anti-inflammatory boost

Pineapples contain a very potent enzyme called bromelain, which has been shown to interrupt the activity of substances that switch on inflammation. Bromelain is found in the highest concentrations in the tougher core of the pineapple, the bit that most people throw away, so make sure you include this. Bromelain has been studied in the context of common inflammatory disorders such as arthritis, with positive findings. It should be noted, however, that the largest proportion of these studies use concentrated extracts, rather than regular culinary doses.

Digestive health

Bromelain in pineapple is a proteolytic enzyme, meaning it can break down proteins. So powerful is this action that it is actually used to tenderize steaks. Some people claim that eating pineapple with protein-based meals aids their digestion.

OTHER BENEFITS
Rich in vitamin C and dietary fibre

BEST WAY TO USE
Eaten fresh or juiced

PLUMS

Plums are one of those fruits that seem to have been overlooked in recent years, in favour of more exotic or lesser-known fruits. But there are many beautiful varieties to try.

GOOD FOR
- Heart health

Heart health

In all of the dark-coloured plums there are high levels of flavonoids. These are part of the chemistry that delivers the dark colour. Flavonoids have been the subject of a great deal of study, particularly here in the UK. They are known to reduce blood pressure by causing the lining of our blood vessels to secrete nitric oxide that relaxes the walls of our vessels and reduces the pressure within them.

Flavonoids are also known to reduce the oxidation of cholesterol – a process that triggers inflammatory damage in the blood vessel walls, which, in turn, kick-starts the process of arterial plaque formation (see page 141).

Finally, they have a high soluble fibre content, which can help to reduce cholesterol, not to mention support digestive health.

OTHER BENEFITS
High vitamin C content, high broad-spectrum antioxidant content

BEST WAY TO EAT
Eaten fresh

POTATOES

The humble potato has had a bit of a bad rap in recent years, especially from the low-carb fraternity. But this humble staple packs a few surprises.

GOOD FOR
➥ Heart health

Heart health

Potatoes aren't the first thing to spring to mind when we think of heart health. A portion of greasy chips doesn't conjure up images of cardiovascular supremacy now, does it? But a compound has been identified in potatoes called kukoamine that has been shown to lower blood pressure. We don't yet have any real insight as to how – such is the nature of nutritional science.

OTHER BENEFITS

The number one source of vitamin C in the UK diet – strange, but true!

BEST WAY TO EAT

Mashed/puréed, boiled, steamed, baked; or, once a week, it HAS to be roast potatoes

PRAWNS (SHRIMP)

Prawns are the most widely eaten seafood there is, and they are popular the world over. Thankfully, they are very nutritious, too!

GOOD FOR
- Skin health
- Immune health

Skin health

Prawns are incredibly rich in two vital minerals: zinc and selenium. Zinc helps regulate the oil-producing glands in the skin – if the skin is too oily or too dry, extra zinc can help balance things out a little. It is also vital for improved wound healing, as it regulates the activity of white blood cells involved in managing infection and healing wounds. Selenium is also involved in wound healing, and in the reduction of inflammation. Prawns are rich in a fat-soluble antioxidant called astaxanthin, which gives them their distinctive pink colour. Astaxanthin accumulates in the fatty layer of the skin, where it can protect against premature ageing and offer some anti-inflammatory activity. All of these things make prawns a great choice for combatting acne, eczema and psoriasis.

Immune health

The high zinc level in prawns makes them a great food for the immune system. Zinc regulates many of the inner workings of white blood cells, the army of the immune system, ensuring they respond to invaders or damaged cells and tissues.

BEST WAY TO EAT
Very lightly cooked, such as sautéed, stir-fried or grilled (overcooking makes them tough)

PUMPKIN (& SUNFLOWER) SEEDS

These moreish little seeds make an ideal between-meal snack, as they are rich in protein, low in calories and dense in nutrients. Sunflower seeds are identical in their nutritional profile.

GOOD FOR
- High cholesterol
- Fungal conditions
- Acne

High cholesterol

Pumpkin seeds are very rich in a compound called beta sitosterol, which is added to those cholesterol-lowering drinks we see advertised so often. It works by blocking the absorption of cholesterol through the gut, and has had vast amounts of clinical research conducted on it.

Fungal conditions

Pumpkin seeds also contain a substance called cucurbitin, which has shown some rather interesting antifungal activity. It is believed to be particularly useful for digestive parasites such as candida. Although I'm sceptical about the huge attention paid to candida in the natural health world, it does occur in some situations and this compound may well be a valid option.

Acne

Pumpkin seeds are very high in zinc, which helps to regulate the activity of the sebaceous glands. This can help to even out oily, acne-prone skin.

BEST WAY TO USE
Eaten fresh, ideally raw

QUINOA

When I first got into eating healthily in the 1990s, quinoa was a strange ingredient that nobody could pronounce and that only appeared in hardcore health-food stores. Now it is everywhere. Even mainstream coffee shops serve quinoa salads!

GOOD FOR
- Blood sugar regulation
- Plant-based protein

Blood sugar regulation

Quinoa is a great grain choice for keeping blood sugar levels stable. Unlike many grains, quinoa has a very high protein content, which means that it takes far longer to digest than other grains. This increased digestion time leads to a gradual drip-feeding of blood sugar rather than a sudden rush. This keeps blood sugar stable.

Plant-based protein

Even though it is totally unjustified, there is a fear that vegans will not get sufficient protein from their diet. All plants contain amino acids, the building blocks of proteins, so a wide intake of plant foods will give you everything that you need. However, should you seek a complete protein source, then quinoa is going to be high up on your list. It is labelled a 'complete' protein, as it contains all nine essential amino acids.

OTHER BENEFITS
Rich in magnesium, manganese, iron and zinc

BEST WAY TO EAT
As an alternative to rice to accompany a curry, chilli, stew, etc.

RASPBERRIES

Raspberries have seen something of a renaissance in recent times, with some really quite ambitious claims being made about them in recent years.

GOOD FOR
- Antioxidant intake
- Weight management?

Antioxidant intake

Raspberries contain significant levels of antioxidants, which can disarm harmful free radicals. These are unstable oxygen particles that can collide into cells and tissues causing them harm, including inflammation and damage to DNA. They are unstable because they lack an electron on their outer surface, and clatter into cells and structures to try to steal an electron to stabilize themselves. Antioxidants disarm free radicals by donating an electron to them. Note that you get more antioxidant bang for your buck when consuming fully ripe raspberries, with up to 50% more in fully ripened raspberries.

Weight management?

One of the reasons that raspberries have suddenly become trendier is due to the discovery of a substance called rheosmin, otherwise known as raspberry ketones. This has made its way into a million and one weight-loss supplements. Some early research has suggested that rheosmin can increase oxygen usage and heat generation in fat cells. This has led to this data being used to draw absolute conclusions that supplementing with raspberry ketones can be a weight-loss aid. It seems that this is jumping the gun a little bit and the studies are in their very early stages. Just eat the fruit as part of a good diet.

OTHER BENEFITS

High in fibre and vitamin C

BEST WAY TO EAT

Whole, juiced or in smoothies

SALMON

We have all heard the recommendation to eat more oily fish due to their multitude of benefits, but many of us are put off by the potent flavour they often have. However, salmon is one that seems to be a popular choice for many and is the most widely eaten oily fish of all.

GOOD FOR
- Heart and circulation
- Inflammatory conditions
- Neurological health

Heart and circulation

Salmon is packed with omega-3 fatty acids, those all-important good fats. These help maintain healthy cholesterol levels and protect the blood vessels from inflammatory damage, which can be the first step in the process that later leads to heart attacks. Omega-3 is also beneficial in regulating the rate and extent to which blood clots.

Inflammatory conditions

Omega-3 fatty acids are very powerful anti-inflammatory agents. The body actually transforms them into our own built-in anti-inflammatories that can 'turn off' the inflammatory reaction.

Neurological health

Omega-3 is also vital for the health of the brain and nervous system. The cells have a special arrangement of fatty material on their outer surface, called the myelin sheath, which is vital for sending and receiving messages. This fatty material can get damaged, and needs adequate essential fats for maintenance.

Research has shown that omega-3 can be beneficial in issues such as depression, memory enhancement and even behaviour and mood stability.

BEST WAY TO EAT
Baked, pan-fried or as a sashimi

SPINACH

Spinach is another of those ingredients that makes its way into almost every savoury dish I concoct.

GOOD FOR
- Skin health

Skin health

Spinach, believe it or not, is a very dense source of carotenoids. We usually associate this with orange- and yellow-pigmented foods, but in spinach, the high levels of green chlorophyll mask the presence of the carotenoids. These fat-soluble antioxidants are the ones that will accumulate in the subcutaneous layer of the skin and protect the structures there from damage.

OTHER BENEFITS
High in vitamin C and magnesium

BEST WAY TO EAT
Eaten raw in salads, juiced, lightly steamed or boiled to retain the nutrients; don't overcook

STRAWBERRIES

Another fruit that is a real British favourite, particularly during the summer. I have great childhood memories of going out strawberry picking and leaving with an empty basket, with strawberry juice all around my face. As well as tasting amazing, they pack a great nutritional punch, too.

GOOD FOR
→ Cardiovascular health

Cardiovascular health

You should by now be starting to see a pattern forming: between berries and heart disease. It is there and it is a prominent one, and strawberries present no exception. They are awash with antioxidant compounds that have been shown to reduce platelet aggregation (clotting), reduced oxidation of triglycerides and vasodilation. One particularly interesting effect they have is to increase the activity of an enzyme called paraoxonase-1 (PON-1). This enzyme can break down particular types of fats that have been oxidized and that can cause significant damage to vessel walls, instigating plaque formation, which can lead to heart disease.

OTHER BENEFITS
High in vitamin C, manganese and fibre

BEST WAY TO EAT
Whole, juiced or in smoothies

SWEET POTATOES

Sweet potatoes have really increased in popularity thanks
to the rise in healthy-eating practices. I remember when I got
into healthy eating around 1992 that they were extremely rare
at that time, and most people would look at them and scratch
their heads. Now they are one of the carbohydrate staples
of the health conscious.

GOOD FOR
- Skin health
- Digestive health
- Immune support

Skin health

As with carrots (see page 147), sweet potatoes contain high
levels of beta carotene, the antioxidant substance responsible
for their bright orange colour. This fat-soluble antioxidant
can begin to accumulate in the fatty subcutaneous layer of
the skin that houses important structures such as the collagen
and elastin fibre matrix that give skin its structural integrity,
suppleness and flexibility. The subcutaneous layer of the skin
also houses the pilosebaceous unit, where the hair follicle and
sebaceous gland meet. By accumulating in the subcutaneous
layer, fat-soluble antioxidants such as carotenoids offer localized
protection to these structures from free radical damage.

Digestive health

Sweet potatoes are very high in fibre, which is the first way
in which they support digestive health. Dietary fibre takes on
many times its own weight in water and swells in the digestive
system. This stretches the gut wall and causes stretch receptors
to stimulate peristalsis, the rhythmical contraction process

that moves the gut contents along efficiently through the various stages.

The second way that sweet potatoes benefit digestive health is due to the substance that gives them their sweet flavour – fructooligosaccharide (FOS). This is a large molecular weight sugar that requires our gut bacteria to break it down. During the breakdown, gut bacteria grow in number and also produce by-products that protect and repair the gut.

Immune support

Some initial studies in China have shown that sweet potatoes contain a type of stored protein, one that the plant uses as a fuel source during various stages of its growth cycle, that can stimulate certain white blood cells within the immune system. The exact mechanisms are not clear, but this interesting first stage of research may lead to further studies down the line.

BEST WAY TO EAT

Roasted, in soups, in curries, grated in röstis

TOMATOES

These are the staple of any salad drawer, and the superstars of the Mediterranean diet. Tomatoes not only taste wonderful, they are little nutritional superstars, too.

> **GOOD FOR**
> ➤ Heart and circulation
> ➤ Prostate health

Heart and circulation

Tomatoes are packed with two important antioxidant nutrients: vitamin C and lycopene. Lycopene is a carotenoid compound responsible for much of the red colour that is important to heart health because it reduces lipid peroxidation, a naturally occurring damage to dietary fats that can cause damage to the blood vessel walls, which then sets the stage for heart disease.

Prostate health

There has been a great deal of research on the link between lycopene and prostate health, and the evidence is mixed. There is, however, some evidence to suggest that populations that consume high levels of lycopene have fewer prostate-related health problems.

OTHER BENEFITS

Tomatoes are also a great source of potassium and vitamin K

BEST WAY TO EAT

Eaten raw or cooked both offer benefits: raw gives you optimal vitamin C levels; cooked makes the lycopene more bioavailable

Common Nutritional Supplements

Nutritional supplements are big business and have become a very popular health choice for those wanting to look after their long-term health. The question often arises, though, as to whether they are necessary. Well, I have mixed views on this. I think it is wise for everyone to take a good-quality multivitamin and essential fatty acids, but the water gets a bit murkier when we start looking at the individual nutrients.

Benefits of a multivitamin

So, why is a multivitamin a good idea? Well, for years we have been told that a varied diet will give us all that we need. It's not that simple, in reality, unless one has the resources and means to eat healthy, diverse food. What's more, we often read that, for example, 100g (3½oz) of broccoli contains X amount of this vitamin, Y amount of that. My response is, 'How do you know?' Many of these nutrients in question are very fragile and their quality depends on the following:

- How fresh the produce is
- How it was harvested
- How it was stored
- How long it was in storage

All of these factors can affect the nutritional value of the produce. Let's use vitamin C as an example. The levels in the crop remain fairly stable while it is growing, but as soon as the crop is harvested, say when an orange is picked, the level of vitamin C immediately starts to decline. If you eat it straight away, all good. If you leave it for three weeks and then eat it, the level of vitamin C has declined massively, and some supermarket produce can be cold stored for months! So, the point is that there is absolutely NO guarantee that the food we eat will contain necessary amounts of these fragile nutrients. On that basis, a good daily multivitamin is a sensible choice, just to ensure the bases are covered.

When it comes to individual nutrients, there is certainly some justification for their use in specific circumstances, such as addressing imbalances and stimulating or manipulating certain biochemical pathways. However, when used improperly, they can do more harm than good. With ready access to all manner of vitamins and nutrients, the general public doesn't know what and what not to take, especially when bombarded by marketers and the media. Taking specific supplements for certain conditions should be done under the care and instruction of a nutritional practitioner, so don't just start taking any old vitamin because you've heard it's good – or all the celebrities are reaping the benefits.

This chapter is here to give you an overview of the most common vitamin, mineral and other types of nutritional supplements on the market and how they can be used, and anything you need to look out for and be aware of.

What this chapter DOESN'T do is replace the advice and care of a nutritional practitioner. In clinic, I would spend an hour with you going through your medical history, perhaps run tests and get an overview of your overall health. This chapter is just a rough guide.

PLEASE NOTE: the nutrients in this chapter are the popular nutritional supplements most people will come across in their health-food store or supermarket.

VITAMINS

Vitamin A

Vitamin A is really a collective name for a group of fat-soluble nutrients called retinoids, which include retinol, retinal and retinyl esters, and the carotenoids. The first, retinol, is essentially what we would call preformed vitamin A that goes straight into use. Retinol is found in animal foods such as liver, red meat and full-fat dairy products.

Carotenoids, such as beta carotene, are sources of vitamin A that are found in plant foods. They make up pigments in plants such as the vivid orange flesh that gives foods like sweet potatoes and carrots their bright orange colour. These forms of vitamin A are complexes. Beta carotene, for example, is two molecules of vitamin A bound head to head, functioning as one entity. If cut in two by enzymes in the body, these molecules form two individual vitamin As.

FUNCTIONS IN THE BODY
- Eye health
- Immune support
- Skin health
- Antioxidant

Eye health

Vitamin A plays a vital role in healthy eyesight. Firstly, vitamin A protects the surface of the eye, the cornea, helping to keep it healthy, and also stops eyes from getting too dry. Beta carotene and lutein (another carotenoid), in particular, have been shown to reduce the risk of macular degeneration – the gradual decline in the health of the macula, the central part of the retina at the back of the eye, that comes from oxidative damage.

Vitamin A also forms part of the rhodopsin molecule that is activated when light hits the retina. Once activated, this molecule sends signals to the brain, resulting in vision. The better this system works, the better we can see, especially in low light conditions such as at night. Have you ever heard the old saying that carrots can help you see in the dark? Well, there is some truth in that!

Immune support

Vitamin A has several important roles to play when it comes to the immune system. For example, it supports the normal growth and regeneration of one of the first barriers of defence against infection: the mucous membranes. These skin-like structures line many organs and tissue surfaces in the body and act as physical barriers to pathogens and harmful substances.

Another role played by vitamin A in immunological support is directly influencing certain lines of white blood cells that act as the army of our immune system. It supports the functioning of neutrophils, macrophages and natural killer cells – types of white blood cells capable of instigating different responses to pathogens and infection.

Vitamin A is also important for the development of T helper cells and B cells – other types of white blood cells that help to orchestrate and regulate the way in which other white blood cells form an attack. They rally the troops, so to speak.

Skin health

Vitamin A is a vital nutrient for healthy skin on many levels. Firstly, the carotenoids can naturally accumulate rapidly in the subcutaneous layer of the skin. This is the fatty layer underneath the skin that contains important structures such as the collagen and elastin fibres that give skin its structural strength, its foundations. Over time, these structures can weaken and be damaged by free radicals – highly reactive chemical substances that can arise from normal metabolic functions, exposure to harmful substances like cigarette smoke, alcohol, etc. Too much time in the sun, smoking cigarettes, pollution, etc. can increase free radical load in the skin. This will chip away at collagen and elastin and weaken it. As these structures get more and more damaged, skin will start to sag, wrinkles will become more deep set and its natural, youthful plumpness will begin to fade. Regularly consuming good sources of beta carotene will help to reinforce the skin's subcutaneous layer. Once in place, it can protect structures like collagen and elastin from free radical damage, offering a long-term, anti-ageing effect.

Vitamin A, particularly the preformed retinoids (retinol, retinal and retinyl esters), appear to reduce the damage caused to skin from ultraviolet radiation (UV rays). It seems they influence some of the biochemical events that take place in the skin upon exposure to ultraviolet light that lead to the breakdown of important tissue structures.

Antioxidant

The carotenoid group of vitamin A compounds have a potent antioxidant effect. They can disarm certain types of free radicals (see above). Carotenoids have a particular affinity for lipid-derived free radicals, meaning ones that come from fatty substances. Top of the list in this category are oxidized cholesterol (i.e. where cholesterol reacts with oxygen and can potentially become toxic) and blood lipids. These can cause untold damage to the endothelium that lines the inside of our blood vessels, setting the stage for plaque formation in the renal arteries, which can lead to heart disease. By reducing the presence of oxidized blood lipids, we can greatly improve our cardiovascular (heart) health.

Who should take vitamin A?

Vitamin A deficiency is very rare indeed, and it is a nutrient that shouldn't be supplemented flippantly. However, patients with acne or very sensitive skin may benefit from a small amount of supplementation.

RECOMMENDED DOSAGE

For men, a dose of around 700mcg per day; women 600mcg daily. Be very careful not to exceed the recommended dose. These levels are perfectly fine, but higher than this over a long period of time can increase the risk of toxicity and liver damage.

SAFETY CONSIDERATIONS

As mentioned, vitamin A is a fat-soluble nutrient group. In the active retinoid forms, it has the potential to become toxic if taken long term in quantities over 1500mcg daily. Beta carotene is not associated with any toxicity. Pregnant women are advised not to take high doses of vitamin A due to the risk of birth defects.

B GROUP

The B vitamin group contains some of the most important nutrients for human health, yet it is B vitamins we are most commonly deficient in. Stress can burn them up at a rate of knots, and they are also water-soluble nutrients, which means that they can soon leach out of the body. Their effects in the body are far-reaching.

FUNCTIONS IN THE BODY
- Important role in metabolism
- Brain health

Vitamin B1 (Thiamin)

Thiamin was the first of the B vitamins to be discovered, and its discovery came about from researching the condition known as beriberi, which arises from B1 deficiency and manifests as confusion, fluid retention, high blood pressure and heart disturbances. In recent years it has become a focal point in research surrounding cognitive function.

Important role in metabolism

Vitamin B1 plays an important role in metabolism. It is involved in the manufacture of adenosine triphosphate (ATP), the fuel that our cells run on made from the glucose that we eat. It is also involved in the breakdown of proteins and fats. Thiamin is particularly known for improving energy production in the brain.

Brain health

Thiamin is an important nutrient for brain health, particularly in the ageing brain. As mentioned, it plays an important role in energy production in the brain, but its benefits go way beyond that. Thiamin seems to empower and also mimic the neurotransmitter acetylcholine, which is involved in memory and learning. Thiamin supplementation has, in several studies, shown some promise for patients suffering with Alzheimer's and dementia.

Who should take thiamin?

As a general rule, B vitamins should always be taken together as a 'B complex', but for some individuals, supplementation with single B vitamins can be useful. Thiamin can be particularly beneficial for students and people who want to optimize their memory and learning. Under clinical supervision, patients with issues around cognitive decline may be suitable candidates.

RECOMMENDED DOSAGE

For most, a daily dose of 50–100mg per day will suffice.

SAFETY CONSIDERATIONS

There are no known toxicity issues with thiamin. As a water-soluble nutrient, any excess is excreted in the urine.

Vitamin B2 (Riboflavin)

This vital B vitamin was discovered back around a century ago. If you are familiar with taking vitamin supplements and have become aware of the unusual side effect that often ensues – the florescent yellow/green urine – you can thank riboflavin for that.

FUNCTIONS IN THE BODY
⬤ Energy production

Energy production

Riboflavin is one of the single most important factors in the production of energy in our cells. When we digest food, we eventually break it down into its most basic of components. Out of these smallest components, the main fuel source is glucose. When glucose enters our cells, it still has to be converted into the one last substance that actually fuels our cells: adenosine triphosphate, or ATP for short (see page 206). This substance is manufactured when glucose enters a cell and moves into a structure within the cell called the mitochondria. When glucose enters the mitochondria, it goes through two stages of chemical transformation: the Krebs cycle, or citric acid cycle (CAC), and the electron transport chain. Riboflavin is responsible for a major part of the Krebs cycle, and insufficient levels of it in our diet can massively inhibit our ability to turn our food into energy, leaving us feeling tired and weak.

Who should take riboflavin?

B vitamins should always be taken as a complex, but extra riboflavin can be a great option for those who need an extra energy boost, or are pushing themselves, be it through athletic endeavours or working life.

RECOMMENDED DOSAGE

50–100mg daily.

SAFETY CONSIDERATIONS

There are no known toxicity issues with riboflavin.

Vitamin B3 (Niacin)

This is one of the most widely distributed B vitamins in the body and it is absolutely vital that we get enough of it.

FUNCTIONS IN THE BODY
- Energy production
- Cardiovascular health
- Skin health

Energy production

Similar to riboflavin, niacin plays a vital role in the Krebs cycle. This is the first stage of the biochemical conversion of glucose into adenosine triphosphate (ATP), within the mitochondria of our cells see page 208).

Cardiovascular health

Niacin can support cardiovascular health in a few ways. Several studies have shown that supplementation with niacin can have positive influences on cholesterol and blood lipids (fats) in three ways in particular: lowering LDL cholesterol ('bad' cholesterol), elevating HDL cholesterol ('good' cholesterol) and lowering triglycerides (see page 83). This triple whammy offers great long-term cardiovascular protection.

The second way in which niacin supports cardiovascular health is at the blood vessel level. It appears that niacin can help to enhance the resilience of the endothelium, the inner skin that lines the insides of blood vessels. By making this surface more resilient to damage, there is less chance of the type of disruption to this surface occurring that can lead to the formation of plaque in the renal arteries, otherwise known as an atheroma.

Niacin in certain forms can also have a vasodilatory function (it can widen blood vessels), helping to lower blood pressure.

Skin health

Niacin is a vitamin that is often prescribed for skin lesions such as acne. This is because it is involved in the management of inflammation. Acne is an infection, so consists of a great deal of inflammation during a flare-up. That angry redness that occurs when spots first break out is inflammation that arises as the immune system responds to the infection. Anything that can ease inflammation will rapidly reduce the severity of the lesion in both feel and appearance.

Who should take niacin?

Niacin is definitely a wise consideration for anyone with a family history of cardiovascular disease or who has high cholesterol and high blood pressure. The beauty of this supplement is that it can be safely taken alongside cholesterol medications.

RECOMMENDED DOSAGE

100mg–500mg daily.

SAFETY CONSIDERATIONS

When taken in the nicotinic acid form, doses of niacin above 400mg can cause rapid flushing of the skin. While this isn't harmful, some people may fund the experience rather unpleasant. Look for 'No-flush niacin'.

Vitamin B5 (Pantothenic Acid)

This vital B vitamin is one of the most widely distributed in our food chain, so deficiency is rare.

FUNCTIONS IN THE BODY
- Cardiovascular health
- Supports cognitive function

Cardiovascular health

Vitamin B5 supports cardiovascular health mainly by its influence on cholesterol. It is involved in cholesterol synthesis, and has been shown to improve LDL/HDL cholesterol ratios, and also lower triglycerides (see page 83).

Supports cognitive function

It has become clear in recent years that all of the B vitamins have vital roles to play in maintaining our long-term cognitive health in numerous ways. Firstly, vitamin B5 is involved in the production of acetylcholine, which plays a role in memory, and also in nerve signal conduction. B5 is also a key nutrient in reducing stress and anxiety, which can give a feeling of enhanced cognitive function when the mind is less overcome with stress and tension.

Who should take vitamin B5?

B5 is found in a very wide variety of foods, so the chances of anyone being deficient in it are slim. In general, I would advise taking a good-quality B complex that contains all of the B vitamins. However, those who have high cholesterol or are worried about heart health may consider additional B5.

RECOMMENDED DOSAGE

50mg–200mg daily.

SAFETY CONSIDERATIONS

There are no known toxicity or safety issues with B5.

Vitamin B6 (Pyridoxine)

Vitamin B6 is one of the most vital B vitamins because of the things that it is directly involved in manufacturing in the body.

FUNCTIONS IN THE BODY
- Cardiovascular health
- Immune support

Cardiovascular health

Vitamin B6 has been a focal point of cardiovascular disease research since 1948. In recent times, this focus has been justified, as it is now known that people with low serum concentrations can have up to a five-times increased risk of heart attack. This may be in part due to the role of B6 in lowering homocysteine – a substance that can cause significant cardiovascular damage and that has long been seen as a marker for heart disease risk.

Vitamin B6 can also reduce platelet aggregation (excess blood clotting). Aggregated platelets in blood vessels can stimulate cellular changes in damaged areas of the vessel walls, which is part of the atheroma (plaque) formation process.

Finally, B6 helps to reduce blood pressure. Excessive pressure against the vessel walls can increase the likelihood of damage to them and the rupture of any current areas of damage, which can cause clots, bleeds and further damage.

Immune support

Vitamin B6 helps to support the immune system in several ways. Low levels of B6 are associated with reduced quality and quantity of antibodies, shrinkage of lymphatic tissues and reduced number and activity of lymphocytes (immune cells).

Who should take vitamin B6?

B6 is present in a very wide variety of plant foods, so a diet with a good selection of fruits and vegetables in it should provide sufficient to prevent deficiency. People may consider a supplement if they have a family history of heart disease or high cholesterol, or have been burning the candle at both ends and want to support their immunity.

RECOMMENDED DOSAGE

50–100mg daily.

SAFETY CONSIDERATIONS

There are no known toxicity issues associated with B6.

Biotin (Vitamin B8)

The B vitamin biotin is one of the most important regulators of metabolism. Metabolism is a word that is used to mean weight management in day-to day-conversation, but metabolism actually means the biological conversion of one thing into another. So this B vitamin is vital in the biological conversion of key substances in the body.

FUNCTIONS IN THE BODY
- Regulates chemical conversion, i.e. metabolism
- Skin, hair and nail health
- Supports blood sugar management

Regulates chemical conversion

As stated, biotin is an essential catalyst in many different reactions that create vital substances in the body. It is a cofactor that is required by several carboxylase enzymes – specific enzymes that help the body to metabolize fatty acids and amino acids. This in itself can influence everything from managing inflammation to stabilizing mood.

Skin, hair and nail health

Biotin has earned the nickname 'the beauty nutrient' because of its influence on the health of skin, hair and nails. Several randomized controlled trials on women with thinning hair have shown an increase in hair thickness and volume when taking biotin supplements. Other studies have found that increased biotin intake can strengthen and harden fingernails. Biotin can also help to reduce flare-ups of skin rashes, eczema and acne.

Supports blood sugar management

Biotin has some important roles to play in the utilization of glucose in the body. Firstly, it enhances insulin sensitivity; insulin is the hormone released by the pancreas when our blood sugar rises. It tells our cells, by way of binding to them, that glucose is available for use, and allows them to take it in and use it for energy. Cells' sensitivity to the signal given by insulin can have a massive impact on blood sugar levels, and many aspects of our modern diet can make us far less sensitive to the insulin signal. This, in the long run, can raise cholesterol and of course increase the risk of type 2 diabetes arising.

The second role biotin plays in blood sugar management is in manufacturing the enzyme glucokinase. This is the enzyme responsible for the first steps of the liver's use of glucose. The liver uses a vast amount of glucose and adequate glucokinase activity can ensure reduced circulating blood glucose, by making sure the liver gets the amount it needs to remain fully fuelled up.

Who should take biotin?

Biotin is a great supplement for anyone wanting to support the health of skin, hair and nails through nutrition, and it has a great safety record.

RECOMMENDED DOSAGE

30–100mcg daily.

SAFETY CONSIDERATIONS

There are no known toxicity issues with biotin.

Folic Acid (Vitamin B9)

Folic acid is likely the most widely known of the B vitamins, or at least the one that people will have heard of, due to its well-documented role in pregnancy.

FUNCTIONS IN THE BODY
- Cell division
- Supports foetal development
- Reduces homocysteine

Cell division

Folic acid is absolutely vital for proper cell division. This can be in times of growth and normal day-to-day maintenance. Its importance is its role in DNA synthesis – the replication of DNA, the master code inside our cells, when the cell is copied. If this process goes wrong, genes can be affected, which may, in turn, lead to severe health problems.

Supports foetal development

The most widely known and discussed benefit of folic acid is its influence on foetal development and the prevention of birth defects. The most well known of these defects are the neural tube defects such as spina bifida. This is where the protective sheath that grows around the spinal cord during development doesn't close properly. This leaves a gap, exposing neurons to potential damage, which can be as severe as paralysis.

In this context, all the evidence points to the requirement of a folic acid supplement before conception or immediately after confirming a pregnancy, as a baby's brain and nervous system begin forming within the first 12 weeks of pregnancy.

Reduces homocysteine

Homocysteine has been discussed previously in this section on B vitamins (see page 214), so I won't labour the point. But it is worth mentioning that high levels of this amino acid metabolite (i.e. the product of a metabolic process or event) have been associated with increased incidence of cardiovascular disease. What isn't clear is whether homocysteine is a causative factor in its own right, as many believe, or whether it is a marker for other pathological processes. Either way, increased intake of key B vitamins, including folic acid, is associated with homocysteine's reduction and a reduction in cardiovascular disease risk.

Who should take folic acid?

This is a supplement with a really strong justification for use pre- and during pregnancy. It is advisable to start taking it as soon as you are planning to become pregnant or as soon as you find out that you are, as many of its key benefits will be realized before the 12-week mark.

RECOMMENDED DOSAGE

400mcg daily.

SAFETY CONSIDERATIONS

There are no known toxicity issues associated with folic acid.

Vitamin B12

Vitamin B12 is another of the B vitamins that has been widely covered in the popular press in recent years, particularly with the explosion of the vegan movement. B12 is the one nutrient that is assumed impossible to obtain on a vegan diet, so there is a long-running debate regarding the potential for vegans to become B12 deficient. This is a very real concern. Many vegans overlook it because the deficiency takes many years to manifest itself. B12 actually pools in the body and this pool can last for anywhere up to six years. So people can eat a B12-deficient diet for many years and not see the signs. However, in time, the effects creep in, fatigue and brain fog being the big signs. At this stage, deficiency is pretty benign. If left to continue, it can evolve into pernicious anaemia, which brings with it intense fatigue and a failure to thrive. Pernicious anaemia occurs when the red blood cells do not form properly and therefore cannot carry oxygen in the way they are meant to. This means tissues cannot meet their oxygen needs and things can break down very quickly.

B12 has also been widely researched in the ageing population, with some quite interesting outcomes being revealed. Ongoing research at Harvard University, for example, has found that B12 supplementation can reduce brain shrinkage and cognitive decline.

FUNCTIONS IN THE BODY
- Prevents pernicious anaemia
- Supports cognitive function

Prevents pernicious anaemia

Pernicious anaemia is a nasty result of long-term vitamin B12 deficiency. The condition can arise from an autoimmune situation, in which the body's immune system attacks its own tissues, causing damage and triggering further disease. Alternatively, pernicious anaemia can arise from restricted intake or absorption of vitamin B12.

Unlike the other B vitamins, B12 can actually pool in the body and be stored for several years, and signs of its deficiency can be slow in coming. Restrictive diets, such as a vegan one, and advancing age can both influence B12 status. B12 comes from animal foods, so vegans do not get exposure to good food sources. In advancing age, even if we eat plenty of B12, our absorption may be impaired. This can be due to two things. Firstly, with advancing age, our secretion of hydrochloric acid (HCL) in the stomach can be reduced. HCL is vital for the release of B12 from food. Also, a substance called intrinsic factor (IF), which binds to B12 to actively assist in its absorption, decreases with age. The production and release of intrinsic factor can also be affected by an autoimmune response that damages the parietal cells – those that secrete intrinsic factor and HCL.

Pernicious anaemia is a type of anaemia that consists of large, immature blood cells forming and entering circulation in place of fully matured healthy ones. Mature red blood cells have four proteins bound to them, creating haemoglobin, which carries oxygen to our tissues.

The large, underdeveloped red blood cells, characteristic of pernicious anaemia, lack haemoglobin, thus their oxygen-carrying capacity is limited. This leads to insufficient oxygen saturation in tissues, which eventually leads to tiredness, fatigue and even numbness and weakness of the hands and feet. In cases of pernicious anaemia, liquid B12 can remedy the condition very rapidly.

Supports cognitive function

B12, like many in the B vitamin group, plays some key roles in the brain that can drastically affect cognitive function.

Firstly, B12 plays an important part in memory, learning and recall, and low levels of this vitamin are found in a high percentage of patients with dementia. In some cases where the dementia isn't full Alzheimer's, B12 supplementation can yield some very positive improvements in memory. There is plausibility behind this, too. With age, we experience a decline in intrinsic factor (IF), which is needed for B12 absorption (see page 221). This, coupled with narrowing dietary choices and variety that often accompany advancing years, means that many older people have significantly reduced B12 intake, which can manifest itself in many ways.

B12 status has also been linked with symptoms of depression, again commonly in the elderly. B12 is a necessary cofactor in the biochemical processes that manufacture neurotransmitters such as the 'feel-good' chemical serotonin.

Who should take vitamin B12?

This is a vital nutrient for vegans to supplement with. There are no plant sources of B12, so deficiency risk is high in those with a plant-based diet. Adults over the age of 50 can also benefit from taking B12, particularly in a liquid form. Patients taking antacid medications, such as omeprazole, can benefit from B12 supplementation due to reduced absorption.

RECOMMENDED DOSAGE

Up to 1000mcg daily.

SAFETY CONSIDERATIONS

There are no known toxicity issues associated with B12.

Vitamin C

This is probably the most well known and widely talked about of the vitamins, and is the number one selling nutritional supplement. It is an essential nutrient to humans. Many animals can actually make this vitamin themselves, but we need to get it from food.

FUNCTIONS IN THE BODY
- Supports immunity
- Antioxidant
- Skin health

Supports immunity

This is one area of vitamin C's function that has been the centre of some debate and controversy, mostly due to its performance in clinical trials for the treatment of the common cold. For several decades now, against the backdrop of the millions of recommendations, there have been studies undertaken to determine whether vitamin C is indeed something of benefit for the common cold, and to say results have been mixed is an understatement. Some trials have shown benefit; others have shown it to be as good as useless.

However, vitamin C certainly DOES have a vital role to play in the immune system. It is used by some lines of white blood cells to deliver the 'oxidative burst'. This is a response by white blood cells when they meet pathogens – a cloud of highly corrosive chemicals released from the cells that smothers the pathogen to kill it.

Vitamin C also has a role to play in assisting the migration of white blood cells to the site of infection.

Antioxidant

Vitamin C is the most important water-soluble antioxidant for our bodies. This means that it is active in watery environments in the body such as the blood, as well as intra- and extra-cellular fluid. As an antioxidant, it means that vitamin C can stabilize highly unstable, and potentially highly reactive, substances that occur naturally in our bodies during normal metabolic functions and produced excessively through cigarette smoking, excessive alcohol consumption, exposure to ultraviolet radiation (UV rays), environmental pollutants, increased stress, etc. These substances are basically missing an electron that they lost during previous chemical reactions, and they go around the body trying to steal one back, colliding into cells and tissues, creating untold damage and potentially triggering disease. Antioxidants such as vitamin C diffuse the situation by 'donating' an electron to these unstable substances.

Vitamin C also helps to recycle vitamin E, which can become spent after delivering its own antioxidant activity (see page 229).

Skin health

Vitamin C helps to reduce the damage done to the skin by UV rays and, in its antioxidant capacity, protects key structures in the skin from UV damage. Exposure to UV radiation depletes vitamin C levels in the skin rapidly, too, which is why we need it.

Vitamin C can also assist in slowing down ageing of the skin. This is because it is vital in the manufacture of collagen – the structural protein that helps skin stay plump and wrinkle free. This structure can become damaged over time with normal ageing processes plus exposure to UV rays, pollutants, cigarette smoke, etc. If the rate of damage exceeds the rate of collagen replenishment (which slows with age), then the skin's structural integrity dwindles, and wrinkles form. Additional vitamin C will assist in collagen replenishment.

Who should take vitamin C?

Vitamin C is very safe and very well tolerated, so almost anyone can use it from time to time. Anyone who spends a lot of time in the sun or maybe burns the candle at both ends (which can affect immunity) may benefit from a supplement.

RECOMMENDED DOSAGE

500mg–1000mg daily.

SAFETY CONSIDERATIONS

Vitamin C has no known serious side effects or toxicity issues. The most widely known adverse effects come from ingesting very high doses (2000–3000mg plus) namely diarrhoea and abdominal cramps. These will pass very rapidly once the excess has left the digestive tract.

Vitamin D

Vitamin D is definitely one of the modern-day nutritional darlings. It was the focus of dozens of studies in the last decade, when new discoveries surrounding its effects and activity were made. It is a nutrient that we can produce naturally in the body. The primary source of vitamin D in humans is the conversion of cholesterol into vitamin D precursors (the substances that then get converted into a vitamin or chemical product) upon exposure to ultraviolet radiation (UV rays). So, as you can imagine, in some parts of the world such as the UK, one can seriously run the risk of deficiency. There are some food sources such as eggs, full-fat dairy and oily fish, but many of us in this part of the world have very low levels in our bodies.

FUNCTIONS IN THE BODY
- Calcium absorption/regulates serum calcium concentrations
- Immune support

Calcium absorption/regulates serum calcium concentrations
Probably the most widely known activity of vitamin D is its influence on the health of the skeleton. People often associate it with the absorption of calcium, but it goes a little further than that. What vitamin D actually does with calcium is two-fold. Firstly, it helps calcium to be absorbed from the gut by stimulating the production of a 'calcium-binding' protein that physically binds to calcium and pulls it across the gut wall and into circulation where it can be put to use. Secondly, vitamin D regulates blood-calcium concentrations. When blood levels get high following absorption from the gut, it shuttles excess calcium into the skeleton and activates cells called osteoblasts that lay down bone and keep the skeleton strong by laying down calcium deposits. Now, we need a certain amount of calcium in

circulation for important functions such as nerve and muscle functions, and if levels start to drop, then vitamin D can activate another group of cells called osteoclasts that break down bone in order to liberate calcium to be sent into circulation to maintain serum concentrations. This is why diets deficient in calcium or vitamin D can become very problematic indeed.

What happens if we are deficient in vitamin D? There are a few known conditions that are related to vitamin D deficiency. The first arises in children: a condition called rickets. Although now very rare in developed countries, there is evidence that it is returning. Rickets is a bowing of weight-bearing bones, particularly in the legs. The bones don't have sufficient hardness from mineralization, so the weight of the growing child upon them causes them to begin to bow and bend and develop deformity. This same softening in adults is called osteomalacia.

Immune support

For decades it was believed that the above activity on the skeleton was all vitamin D was about. However, in recent years we have discovered that it has many more potential roles to play. One area that it is proving beneficial is in supporting the function of the immune system. Vitamin D receptors are found on the B cells, T cells and antigen-presenting cells (APC) of the immune system. These cells can create the active form of vitamin D, too, which is testament to its vital importance in this system. Its activity here appears to be one of 'priming' certain cells to get them ready for action. In essence, it helps to regulate specific responses. There also seems, from early research at least, that there may be some promise for its use in the treatment of autoimmune conditions, as vitamin D may cause the immune system to shift away from this kind of response.

Who should take vitamin D?

I believe there is a solid argument for most inhabitants of Northern Europe to take vitamin D during the winter months, as our exposure is so poor. Anyone with a low calcium intake (who consumes little or no dairy), a family history of osteoporosis and maybe even those with autoimmune conditions should consider vitamin D supplementation.

RECOMMENDED DOSAGE
200–500 IU daily.

SAFETY CONSIDERATIONS
As a fat-soluble nutrient, excessive vitamin D intake can be potentially toxic in long-term doses beyond those described above. Some of the less-serious side effects include weight loss and frequent urination. However, when things take a more serious turn, toxicity can become very dangerous: it can raise calcium concentrations in the blood drastically, which can lead to calcification and hardening of tissues that can damage the heart, blood vessels and kidneys.

Vitamin E

Vitamin E is one of the most widely commercially used vitamins, particularly in the cosmetics industry. It has vital roles to play in our body, some that save our lives daily.

FUNCTIONS IN THE BODY
- Antioxidant
- Potential cardiovascular protection

Antioxidant

Vitamin E is probably best known for its role as an antioxidant. It has a particular affinity for lipid (fat)-derived free radicals and for protecting fatty structures from free radical damage. So vital in this role is vitamin E that it is actually incorporated into the cell membranes in all of our cells. Here it protects this vital structure and its components from damage against free radical attack. This has potential benefits for nearly every single system and tissue in the body, from preventing skin damage and reducing the signs of ageing, to reducing excessive tissue damage throughout the body.

Potential cardiovascular protection

Vitamin E has long had a reputation for being essential to a healthy cardiovascular system, especially due to its antioxidant activity. One of the processes responsible for the early stages of heart disease is the oxidation of cholesterol and triglycerides (blood fats). When they oxidize, they can begin to cause damage to the inner surface of our blood vessels. When this happens, the body responds and tries to repair the damage, and that's when a 'plaque' or 'atheroma' is formed. Preventing damage to the vessel walls helps to minimize plaque formation, and prevents damage and rupture to plaques that are already present.

Another potential way in which vitamin E can offer cardiovascular protection is by interacting with clotting factors – the things that regulate the rate and extent to which blood clots. Clot formation can be fatal. When a clot forms, it can travel through the cardiovascular system, entering smaller and smaller vessels, from arteries to capillaries. Eventually, if it stays intact, it can reach a vessel that is too small to accommodate it, and it can block that vessel. If this happens to a vessel in the heart, a heart attack ensues. If this happens in the brain, it is a stroke.

Who should take vitamin E?

Vitamin E is, in essence, safe in the lower doses. However, in higher doses it is unsuitable for anyone taking anticoagulant medication (blood thinners) such as warfarin. It can be beneficial for anyone in lower doses as part of a multivitamin or daily antioxidant formula.

RECOMMENDED DOSAGE
400 IU daily.

SAFETY CONSIDERATIONS
Vitamin E can have serious interactions with some medications. Blood thinners such as warfarin and aspirin are among the most serious. As vitamin E reduces the activity of clotting factors, when coupled with anticoagulant medications it can deliver a high risk of haemorrhage. There is also some concern regarding taking vitamin E while undergoing chemotherapy, as it may offer some degree of protection to the target cancer cells.

MINERALS

The importance of minerals for human health is often overlooked in the mainstream. Everyone knows about vitamins and antioxidants, but ask them about minerals or trace elements and they often look blank. Minerals are some of the most vital micronutrients for our health. They regulate cellular communication and electrical impulses in the heart and nervous system, and provide structural support, to name but a few functions.

Calcium

Calcium is the best known of all the minerals, and is the most abundant one in the body, making up to 1.5–2% of total body weight, with 99% of that being within the bones.

FUNCTIONS IN THE BODY
- Bone mineralization
- Cell signalling
- Muscle function

Bone mineralization

Maintaining bone mineralization is possibly the most widely known role that calcium has to play in the body. Calcium is the dominant structural material within the bones, alongside phosphorous and magnesium, and is laid down over a soft, criss-cross matrix. Calcium is delivered to the skeleton by vitamin D, which then stimulates cells called osteoblasts to take the calcium and build it into the skeleton. The skeleton can be seen as a calcium bank as well as a structural frame. When blood calcium levels get low, cells called osteoclasts, upon receiving signals from vitamin D, liberate some calcium from the skeleton into the blood.

Cell signalling

Calcium is one of the single most vital substances for cell signalling – cells communicating within the body. Calcium ions move in and out of our cells in accordance to the cells' needs. When required, ion channels in the cell membrane open up to allow calcium ions (and others) inside the cell. Once inside the cell, calcium can regulate the activity of numerous enzymes and proteins that catalyze all manner of reactions.

This is why the body will release calcium from skeletal stores if blood concentrations get too low, because it is so important to so many cellular functions that to be without enough could be disastrous.

Muscle function

Calcium has a fascinating and absolutely essential role to play in muscular contraction. Muscles contract when two neighbouring fibres grab hold of each other and slide along each other. To do this, the neighbouring fibre needs to latch on to a specialized binding site on the fibre next to it. These binding sites are occupied by a substance called tropomyosin while the muscles are relaxed. As soon as a nervous impulse signals the muscles to contract, calcium rushes in and removes the tropomyosin, exposing the binding site, allowing the neighbouring fibre to attach to it, slide it along and contract the muscle.

Who should take calcium?

Calcium is very widely available in the diet, so the chances of reaching a deficiency state are very slim indeed. However, those with a history of osteoporosis should consider supplementing with calcium alongside vitamin D. The only thing to be wary of is not to take the calcium carbonate form, as this is just chalk and is very poorly absorbed by the body. Aim for a higher-quality form like dicalcium malate or calcium citrate.

RECOMMENDED DOSAGE

1000–1200mg daily.

SAFETY CONSIDERATIONS

Excessive calcium intake can lead to a state called hypercalcaemia, which can damage the kidneys and cause calcification of the heart, blood vessels and soft tissues. Calcium supplements can also reduce the effectiveness of the following drugs: bisphosphonates, fluoroquinolone and tetracycline antibiotics, levothyroxine, phenytoin and tiludronate disodium.

Iron

Iron is an absolutely essential element to human life, and deficiency can have immensely negative consequences for our health.

FUNCTION IN THE BODY
➼ Oxygen transport

Oxygen transport

The primary function of iron in the body is to transport oxygen to our tissues. On the surface of our red blood cells we have four proteins bound together to form a structure called haemoglobin. On each of these proteins within haemoglobin, there are sites where iron attaches. Iron then in turn binds to oxygen. When oxygen enters our body from the lungs, it binds to the iron on the haemoglobin, and the red blood cells carry it around the body, depositing it to cells and tissues that need it.

Deficiency in iron leads to the condition known as anaemia. This can manifest itself with tiredness and muscle weakness, and general lack of energy. Sufferers can also experience shortness of breath and heart palpitations, and often present with paleness of the skin.

Who should take iron?

Women often have higher requirements for iron than men due to menstrual blood loss. I often advise women to supplement with iron one week prior to their period and also during it, stopping the supplement when the period ceases.

RECOMMENDED DOSAGE

15–20mg once daily. It is worth noting here, however, that the form that you take it in makes all the difference. The cheap, 'ferrous sulphate' version, often given on prescription, can cause bad constipation. Instead, opt for a form known as iron bisglycinate or 'gentle iron'.

SAFETY CONSIDERATIONS

Iron is one nutrient that has to be treated with extreme caution, and dosages above the recommendations here should never be entertained. Dosages above 30mg daily can begin to displace other minerals and cause false deficiency signs of those nutrients, which will come with its own set of problems. In very large dosages, it can cause organ failure and death, particularly in children, so keep supplements out of their reach. Iron supplementation can reduce the effectiveness of the drug levothyroxine.

Magnesium

Magnesium is one of the most abundant minerals in the body, and one of the most broadly used substances.

FUNCTIONS IN THE BODY
- Enzyme activity
- Energy production
- Cardiovascular health

Enzyme activity

Magnesium is involved in over 1,000 chemical reactions in the body, with over 300 of those being enzyme-driven reactions that occur almost consistently. Enzymes are proteins that facilitate chemical reactions. Magnesium regulates the activity of enzymes, allowing them to function properly and drive their reactions.

Energy production

Magnesium plays an absolutely vital role in the production of energy at a cellular level. When we break food down and release the glucose from it, it enters the cell but still has to be converted into one final product that we can actually use as an energy source, namely adenosine triphosphate (ATP; see page 206). Magnesium affects ATP in two ways: firstly, it has vital roles to play in the first stage of ATP production, the Krebs cycle (see page 208); secondly, magnesium influences ATP by binding with it to form MgATP, which powers up other chemical reactions within cells.

Cardiovascular health

Magnesium is an essential nutrient for the health of the entire cardiovascular system. It has a role to play in regulating heart rhythm and has been used successfully to treat cardiac arrhythmia. It also helps to strengthen the contraction of heart muscles, which is useful in the prevention or management of cardiomyopathy (diseases of the heart muscle) and heart failure. There have been some studies that have shown magnesium to have value in lowering blood pressure. This may be due to its ability to relax smooth muscle, which helps the vessel to dilate and the pressure within it to drop.

Who should take magnesium?

Magnesium is one of the most deficient nutrients in the developed world. It is one of those supplements that anyone could benefit from taking. Its diverse importance and low toxicity means that most of us living fast-paced, stressful lives would do well to take this.

RECOMMENDED DOSAGE

400–1000mg with food, daily. For sleep, take with your evening meal.

SAFETY CONSIDERATIONS

Very high levels of magnesium can cause mild diarrhoea, but this does pass quickly. Some antibiotics, such as tetracycline, can become less effective when taken at the same time as magnesium supplements.

Selenium

Selenium is the most widely supplemented trace mineral (minerals we only need tiny amounts of). It is part of the enzyme glutathione peroxidase (GPx). Glutathione peroxidases are a family of antioxidants also known as selenoproteins.

FUNCTION IN THE BODY
- Glutathione peroxidase (intracellular antioxidant) cofactor

---

Glutathione peroxidase (intracellular antioxidant) cofactor
The primary role that selenium plays is to become part of one of the body's own in-built antioxidant enzymes called glutathione peroxidase. This powerful antioxidant protects cells and cell membranes from oxidative damage, and as such has relevance for many areas of health.

There are links between reduced glutathione peroxidase activity and cardiovascular disease protection, and part of the pathological process of cardiovascular disease is inflammation and oxidation. Glutathione peroxidase can target both. Oxidation of lipids (fats), such as cholesterol and triglycerides, can cause potent damage to blood vessel walls, creating patches of damaged tissue that need repairing, and it is during this repair process that plaque formation occurs. Glutathione peroxidase, carotenoids, vitamin E and omega-3 all help to buffer and reduce this.

Many studies have gone on to influence organizations such as the National Research Council (US) Committee on Diet and Health to determine that selenium has a protective role against cancer, and some even argued in the US for foods to be fortified with selenium. Free radicals have the capacity to cause drastic cellular damage. When they damage cells, they can damage genetic material within the DNA strands in the cell. If this happens, genes that regulate cellular replication may be affected, and cell division may suddenly begin to go haywire and cancer risk goes up. Of course, there are thousands of potential cancer risk factors, but increasing our body's own production of one of its defence mechanisms is a step we can take to have some strength in our corner at least.

Who should take selenium?
Selenium is frequently deficient, so is worthy of inclusion in any multivitamin supplement.

RECOMMENDED DOSAGE
200mcg daily.

SAFETY CONSIDERATIONS
Excess intake of selenium can cause clinical selenosis, which can manifest itself in hair and nail loss, skin lesions and rashes, fatigue, irritability, nausea and diarrhoea.

Zinc

Zinc is found in every single cell in the body. It is an important component of over 200 different enzymes.

FUNCTIONS IN THE BODY
- Immune support
- Supports a healthy pregnancy
- Skin health
- Supports male sexual function

Immune support

While supplements such as vitamin C have at best had mixed results in trials as a remedy for the common cold, zinc has fared far better. Zinc is used by our white blood cells, the foot soldiers of the immune system, to code genes that essentially control the way in which these cells respond to pathogens that they encounter and the types of responses they deliver.

Zinc also has antiviral properties in its own right.

Supports a healthy pregnancy

Zinc is an essential nutrient for proper cell division and as such plays a vital role in foetal development. Low zinc levels in the mother have been linked to premature birth, low birth weight and poor growth rates.

Skin health

Zinc can benefit the health of the skin in two main ways. Firstly, it helps to regulate sebaceous secretions – the production of oil in the skin. If the skin is too oily, then adequate zinc intake can reduce sebum production, making the skin less oily. Conversely, if the skin is too dry, then adequate zinc intake can increase sebum secretion to balance moisture levels in the skin.

The other way that zinc can benefit the skin is in relation to acne. As described previously, zinc is a powerful tool in fighting infection. As acne is an infection of the pilosebaceous unit, supporting the immune system can clear this infection faster.

Supports male sexual function

Zinc is vital for almost every aspect of male sexual function. Low levels of zinc are known to cause a drop in testosterone, and zinc is essential for its manufacture and metabolism. Zinc is also vital for sperm count and how it moves.

Who should take zinc?

Zinc should be a regular part of men's supplement programmes. This becomes more important after age 30, in particular. There is also great evidence for pregnant women to supplement their diet with zinc.

RECOMMENDED DOSAGE

Men: 15–30mg daily. **Women:** 15mg daily.

SAFETY CONSIDERATIONS

Zinc can deliver acute and chronic toxicities. Acute toxicity tends to present as powerful nausea, appetite loss, abdominal cramps and stomach upsets. Chronic zinc toxicity tends to involve upsetting other enzymes, which results in false deficiency signs of other minerals. There have also been some reports of damage occurring to the urinary tract in some individuals.

MISCELLANEOUS

This section is for those few supplements that so many of you may have heard of and that are frequently discussed, but don't fit into the vitamin or mineral categories.

Coenzyme Q10

Coenzyme Q10 (CoQ10) is a vital substance for the correct functioning of our mitochondria – the energy factories inside our cells. CoQ10 also delivers some antioxidant activity.

FUNCTIONS IN THE BODY
- ATP production
- Supports heart health

ATP production
ATP (adenosine triphosphate) is the energy currency that our body runs on. The energy released from the food we eat enters our cells where it goes through two major chemical events that fuel the production of ATP: the Krebs cycle (see page 208) and the electron transport chain. It is in this second stage that CoQ10 is absolutely vital. Users of CoQ10 report noticing a considerable energy boost from taking it.

Supports heart health
CoQ10 offers great long-term support to the health of the heart – again, mostly via ATP production. If you think about it, your heart is the most active muscle of all across your lifespan. It never ceases. The energy requirements this relentless muscle have are immense. In time, however, all of our cells become less effective at making ATP. Additional CoQ10 can keep the heart

making ATP effectively. It also plays a role in keeping all cells stable against free radical attack.

CoQ10 is so efficient at supporting energy production in heart muscle cells that, under clinical supervision, it has been used to treat heart failure. When the heart muscle is weakened and cannot fully and effectively pump blood around the body, serious medical situations begin to arise. CoQ10 can act what is called 'inotropically', meaning that it strengthens the forcefulness of the contraction of the heart muscle. The increased contraction can add an extra bit of oomph and strength to the heart's pumping ability.

Who should take CoQ10?

CoQ10 is great for anyone that needs an energy boost, and for those of us that are at the 40-plus mark. CoQ10 is an ESSENTIAL supplement for statin users. This cholesterol-lowering drug also lowers the levels of the carrier that transports CoQ10 around the body, making it less widely distributed and less available. This can cause symptoms such as weakness, muscle pains, breathlessness and fatigue.

RECOMMENDED DOSAGE
200mg daily.

SAFETY CONSIDERATIONS
There are no known interactions or safety consideration surrounding CoQ10.

Glucosamine

Glucosamine is one of the biggest-selling and most recommended supplements on earth for all things related to joint damage and wear and tear.

FUNCTION IN THE BODY
- Replenishes cartilage

Replenishes cartilage

Glucosamine is a very simple molecule of glucose bound with an amine group. Within the joints, the role of glucosamine is to produce glycosaminoglycans, one of the key structural components of cartilage. As we age, our production of these begins to decline, which causes our cartilage to have less shock-absorbent potential. This makes it more exposed to damage and, in time, the cartilage can break down, leading to osteoarthritis. Supplementing with glucosamine can help to slow down or even improve this.

Who should take glucosamine?

Anyone with cartilage damage, joint pain or osteoarthritis.

RECOMMENDED DOSAGE

This is a dose-dependent nutrient and some of it gets lost in digestion. Aim for at least 1500mg daily.

SAFETY CONSIDERATIONS

There are no known safety issues surrounding glucosamine.

Omega-3 Fatty Acids

Omega-3 fatty acids have become very popular in recent years and are something I am rather obsessed with. Their popularity is immensely justified, in my opinion.

FUNCTIONS IN THE BODY
- Regulates inflammation
- Improves blood fats and cholesterol
- Maintains healthy eyes
- Supports a healthy nervous system

Regulates inflammation

Essential fatty acids such as the omega-3 are metabolic building blocks for structures and substances in the body. One of the key things they help to build is a group of communication compounds called prostaglandins that regulate the inflammatory response. There are different types of prostaglandins, some that turn inflammation on, and some that turn inflammation off. The omega-3 fatty acids EPA and DHA create the types of prostaglandin that switch inflammation off. By increasing omega-3 fatty acids we can reduce inflammation. This can have benefits for nearly every conceivable aspect of health. It can protect us from heart disease, many cancers, ease inflammatory conditions such as arthritis and injuries and even slow down the ageing of the brain.

Improves blood fats and cholesterol

One area in which omega-3 has a very good reputation is improving cholesterol ratios. The two lipoproteins that shuttle cholesterol around the body – LDL and HDL – are often considered bad and good respectively because of the way they deal with cholesterol. LDL is considered bad because it takes cholesterol away from the liver out into the body, and HDL is considered good because it takes cholesterol from the peripheries of the body and brings it back to the liver for recycling. Think of LDL and HDL as two different bus routes. While this metaphor maybe somewhat simplistic, there certainly IS a strong link between higher HDL and reduced risk of heart attack. Omega-3 fatty acids have long been known to reduce LDL and increase HDL.

Maintains healthy eyes

One of the omega-3 fatty acids, DHA, is found in very high concentrations within the retina and is vital for its function, both in development and throughout adult life. This is the area of the eye that receives light and converts it into neural signals, which are sent to the brain for recognition.

Maintains a healthy nervous system

Omega-3 fatty acids, DHA in particular, are a vital part of an important fatty structure that surrounds our nerve cells called the myelin sheath. This specialized structure envelops the core of the nerve in short, capsule-like pieces with tiny gaps of exposed nerve between each one. These exposed gaps are called the nodes of Ranvier, or myelin-sheath gaps. This arrangement allows electrical impulses to jump along nerves at an accelerated rate. This structure is susceptible to environmental damage such as that caused by free radicals, and any damage to it can drastically affect the efficiency of the nerve, so the body constantly rebuilds myelin as it gets damaged. It is essential that we take in sufficient DHA to support remyelination.

Who should take omega-3?

This is one supplement I personally would put the entire nation on. Its potential benefits are hugely significant for everyone, and it is a nutrient that so few of us get anywhere near enough of.

RECOMMENDED DOSAGE

Look for a once-daily supplement that contains around 750mg EPA and 250mg DHA.

SAFETY CONSIDERATIONS

The only real safety considerations around omega-3 are for people on very high dose anticoagulants (blood thinners) such as warfarin. For these cases, alternate-day supplementation will suffice.

INDEX

RESOURCES

Want to work in food, health, and wellness? Want to study
without rigid time commitments and without breaking the bank?

Consider studying at Dale Pinnock's
THE CULINARY MEDICINE COLLEGE

- Evidence based, applied, and practical.
- Study anywhere, anytime. Fit the course around your life.
- No tight deadlines or timescales, take as long as you want.
- Encourages your creativity and teaches you how to build recipes
  around the science with confidence.
- Developed by one of the country's leading voices in nutrition and health.

Accredited and CPD registered.
Our 'Diploma in Culinary Medicine' has been accredited by the CMA
and the FNTP, and has been awarded a value of 5 CPD points to qualified
NTs by the FNTP
www.culinarymedicinecollege.com

DIABETES UK

Diabetes UK is the most widely
known diabetes organization in the
UK. Their website is a great resource
for information on diabetes and
its management.
diabetes.org.uk

BRITISH HEART FOUNDATION

This is probably the best known
organization championing heart health.
Their website is a great resource for
everything from statistics and medical
breakthrough information, through
to practical everyday tips for looking
after your heart.
bhf.org.uk

BRITISH DIETETIC ASSOCIATION

The BDA have developed a great deal
of factsheets that are available for free.
These factsheets comprise information
about specific illnesses/disorders/
system health. They also offer advice
on dietary changes etc.
bda.uk.com/foodfacts/hypertension

VIRIDIAN

Produces over 200 award-winning
supplement products including
vitamins, minerals, herbs, nutritional
oils, speciality supplements, tinctures
and balms. Sold in stockists in over a
dozen countries and ships worldwide
from their online shop.
viridian-nutrition.com